HEALTHY
AT
100

7 Steps
to a Century
of Great Health

Robert D. Willix Jr., M.D. *362 0724*

D0683530

SHOT TOWER BOOKS
Boca Raton, Florida

Printed in the United States of America

Senior Editor: Mark Ford
Managing Editor: Katie Yeakle
Production Editor: Kimberlee Lansdale
Copy Editor: Judith Strauss
Contributing Editors: Kieran Doherty, Denise Foley, and Eileen Nechas
Illustrator: Eve Tanselle
Cover Designer: Pearl Lau

Published by:
    Shot Tower Books, Inc.
    150 East Palmetto Park Road
    Suite 320
    Boca Raton, Florida 33432

ISBN 0-9639629-0-6 softcover

Distributed in the book trade by Atrium Publishers Group

*This book is dedicated
to my wife, Donna Lee ("The Blonde"),
whose continuous love and support
always make a work project
a source of enjoyment.
Thank you for your love!*

Acknowledgments

I would like to express my gratitude to all who have contributed to the writing of this book. I am sure that the reader has no concept of how much of an effort is put forth by so many people in the background to bring these words to a printed format. So, for both the reader and myself, I express my heartfelt appreciation.

If it were not for Mark Ford and his belief in my approach to health, this project would have never gotten off the ground. To all the people at Agora Inc. and Shot Tower Books who have read, reread, and edited the manuscript, I thank you.

I hope that I don't exclude anyone, but, I would like to take this opportunity to name a few of the key contributors who made this book possible — William Bonner, Mark Ford, Katie Yeakle, Kimberlee Lansdale, Judith Strauss, Kathleen Peddicord, and Kieran Doherty.

The final book would never have gotten to this level of professional quality without the tireless efforts of Kimberlee Lansdale, with her meticulous concern for accuracy and detail, and the final touches of the copy editor, Judith Strauss. A very special thanks to both of you for making this a book that we can be proud of.

I also want to thank all of my teachers throughout my life who have challenged me to go beyond my comfort zone and to seek a higher level of knowledge by raising my consciousness.

And thanks to my readers for recognizing that the future of health is a balance between the science of the West and the tradition of the East.

God bless all of you!

Foreword

by Dr. Barry Sears

True health care reform has nothing to do with the increased availability of MRI scans or cheaper health insurance. It begins when an individual finally begins to take responsibility for his or her own health, instead of abdicating that responsibility to a third party. Dr. Willix has provided a state-of-the-art "how-to" guide to reach that goal in this very user-friendly book.

Dr. Willix's program is designed to orchestrate a vast array of powerful hormonal responses that have evolved over the past 40 million years. Don't be misled by his seemingly simple recommendations. Each step, if properly followed, leads to profound, fundamental, physiological changes that everyone can achieve.

Many of the ancient verities of medicine can now be explained by understanding how they operate at the hormonal level to positively affect how the body functions. Understanding the hormonal responses induced by exercise, stress reduction, and diet is the next medical frontier. Eventually, triggering these responses will be considered the primary treatment for all disease states, with drugs being used as secondary backup. Once these chemical effects are finally understood by the medical establishment, a paradigm shift in the practice of medicine will occur.

Obviously, this will not happen overnight. It requires a substantive educational effort to develop a common language that eventually ties together observations from the earliest days of recorded history with the most recent advances in medicine. Without that common language, a medical Tower of Babel is created that prevents a consistent, total approach to wellness.

This book deals with very complex biochemical concepts. Yet, the power of Dr. Willix's program is that anyone can begin to tap into this hormonal control technology simply by following his seven steps. However, to do so, you must take charge of your life by making the time to continually renew your body using this technology. If you don't, you will never reach optimum health, let alone wellness.

"Reaching optimal health" is simply another way of saying "maximizing the quality of your life." Your ultimate goal is not really to reach 100, but to squeeze every bit out of life within your allotted time on this planet. Dr. Willix gives you the rules and the tools to achieve that goal. But only you can initiate their use.

— August 1994

Dr. Sears is a former research scientist at the Boston University School of Medicine and the Massachusetts Institute of Technology. He is currently the president of Surfactant Technologies Inc., a biotechnology company in Marblehead, Massachusetts, specializing in the development of intravenous drug delivery systems for cancer chemotherapy and cardiovascular disease treatment.

Table of Contents

Introduction

by Dr. John Douillard

In this fascinating book, Dr. Willix shows us how simple it is to live up to our human potential. Though our society typically considers life spans of 125 years to be impossible — or possible only for members of exotic societies hidden away in remote, nearly unreachable parts of the world — Dr. Willix shows us how to bring the reality of longevity right into our own lives.

It is no secret that we are functioning at a fraction of our capabilities — mentally and physically. Researchers tell us that we use only about one one-hundredth of one percent of our full potential. We accomplish this undistinguished feat through a lifestyle fraught with exhaustion and stress. We typically push ourselves to the point of collapse in a relentless, neverending drive to do and have more. Obviously, this approach to life cannot provide a sense of happiness or well-being.

Dr. Willix not only paves the way for us to remove such stressors from our lives, he also shows us how to change our ways so that we don't incur the stressors in the first place. The amazing result is that Dr. Willix shows us how to extend our life spans (which is the hallmark of this book), while he shows us how to dramatically improve the quality of life in terms of health and happiness. And this is of major importance. After all, no one wants to live a long life in a barely functional state, farmed out to a nursing home.

After reading this book, you will not fear the future. Rather, you will see it as a time to gracefully age, full of energy and in good health, sharing the wisdom of a lifetime with your children and grandchildren.

In our society, the deterioration that we equate with old age has made us lose respect for those who, in traditional cultures, have always been the most highly revered. As we learn how to be healthy at 100, the dignity of growing old will be restored to us. With that, the elders of our society will regain their rightful place as our leaders.

In *Healthy at 100*, Dr. Willix has blended the scientific findings of the West with the ancient wisdom of the East — where old age is still venerated — better than anyone I have yet seen. He uses scientific proofs as well as centuries-old evidence from other cultures to make an incredibly good case for our potential to extend the current human life span. And he recognizes that today, an intelligent approach to longevity has to include an understanding of the modern lifestyle, plus everything that modern researchers have learned about exercise and nutrition, along with the time-honored techniques of the Orient.

The ancient wisdom that Dr. Willix draws upon has passed the test of time. Ayurvedic medicine, for example, is one of the oldest systems of medicine in the world. Not only that, it is today, as we speak, also one of the biggest. Over 300,000 Ayurvedic practitioners belong to the All Indian Ayurvedic Congress, while the American Medical Association has only about 250,000 doctors as members. And traditional Chinese medicine is still the mainstay of the medical system in China, the largest country in the world.

Dr. Willix reminds us that the world is a huge place with a vast reservoir of knowledge. That the Western way is not the only way, and that there is something for us to learn from all systems of medicine still being practiced today — the biggest and the oldest, as well as the newest and most highly technical. In *Healthy at 100*, he has connected all this information, and has demystified the ancient wisdom by validating it with modern scientific studies.

What Dr. Willix has created here is a must read for people of all ages. His premise is prevention — the prevention of disease and debility — and that it's never too early to begin or too late to start enjoying life. If you follow the prescription that Dr. Willix sets forth in this book, you will be effortlessly charting a positive course for the rest of your life.

— August 1994

*Dr. Douillard is the author of **Body, Mind and Sport** and the "Invincible Athletics" tape series. He is currently in private Ayurvedic practice in Boulder, Colorado.*

21st Century Medicine: Where East Meets West

This is a book about you and your health. But it is unlike any other health book you have ever read.

In the pages of this book, I will give you information that will make it possible for you to cast aside all your old beliefs about age and aging, about illness and pain, and about the eventual, inevitable decay of your own body.

I will also teach you how to take seven easy steps to stop the aging process in its tracks and even, in many cases, reverse it.

The basis of my seven-step program

My seven-step program is based on a marriage between the very latest in modern medical research and the ancient healing arts of India and China — a medical tradition that is older, by thousands of years, than the practice of Western medicine.

This marriage between ancient and modern draws upon my

knowledge of yoga, acupuncture, transcendental meditation, and, most particularly, Ayurvedic medicine (with its understanding of the link between mind and body), and combines these Eastern practices with my expertise in modern technology and Western medicine's more pragmatic or matter-based approach to healing.

The union between East and West, between ancient and modern, has led me to what can only be called a "revolution" in the practice of medicine — a revolution potentially more important than any other medical or scientific event in history. (After all, it deals with life itself!) As a result of this revolution, the practice of medicine is already undergoing rapid changes and will, in just a few years, be vastly different from medicine as we have known it in the latter years of the 20th century.

How different will 21st century medicine be?

The 21st century will witness a new relationship between doctor and patient. A relationship in which the physician — aware of the inviolable link between mind and body — pays as much attention to each patient's emotional health as to his or her physical health. A relationship in which the doctor helps each patient lead a better, fuller, more vibrant and exciting life — a life in which each day can be lived more fully, free of pain, free of fatigue, and full of vitality at any age.

In the 21st century, doctor and patient will form a healing partnership in which the doctor, having learned from his brother and sister healers in the Orient, urges his patients to use meditation, yoga, and relaxation to foster overall well-being. A partnership in which patients are not just health-care "consumers," but are active, vital participants in their own wellness.

Here are just a few of the things that will almost certainly be commonplace in the medical world in the decades to come:

- Meditation and other relaxation techniques will be widely accepted as a way to reduce stress and as a source of power to boost the immune system.
- Vitamins and nutrients (sometimes in very large doses) will play a central role as disease-preventive agents and as guards against the ravages of age.
- Physical fitness will be achieved more through a regimen of moderate exercise than through the high-intensity work-

outs of the past.

- The flu will be a one-day illness instead of the two-week misery we've been used to.
- Osteoporosis, one of the great killers of post-menopausal women, will be a thing of the past.
- Senility will be a forgotten illness.
- Men and women will expect to enjoy their sexual lives no matter how old they become.
- Prostate and colon cancer will be almost completely preventable.
- Death by lung cancer will be uncommon.
- Many 80-year-olds will be stronger than 30-year-olds are today.
- Surgical procedures that are commonplace today will be viewed like medieval tortures.
- "Middle age" will begin at 60 or 70 years of age ... and men and women in their 90s will be leading active, even athletic lives.
- We will live in complete freedom from the expectation that we're destined to die at age 70 ... or 80 ... or even 90. We will live in a world in which we'll expect to live a full, constructive life, free of debilitating illness, for a century or more!

Freedom to become fully alive

Ultimately, 21st century medicine is all about freedom — freedom from the chains of time — freedom from a life circumscribed by disease, aging, pain, and death — freedom to become fully alive with mind-body health!

The secrets of just how this will be possible — secrets more valuable than any others — are what I will reveal to you in this book. In the following pages, I'll teach you what I have learned during the past two decades, first as a physician and a cardiac surgeon, then as a proponent of a new brand of medicine in which diet and exercise are of paramount importance, and most recently as a practitioner of what I choose to call "21st century medicine."

If you make a decision to follow the suggestions and recommendations that I will present to you in the next 200-or-so pages, you will completely transform your life. You can expect — no matter how old you are when you start this program — to live healthfully, with energy and optimism in abundance. You can expect to live without constant or undue pain. And any preconceptions you may have had about the inevitability of getting slower, weaker, or sicker as you age will vanish.

A prescription for healthy longevity

While writing this book, I came across a newspaper column written by Ellen Goodman in which she bemoaned the fact that medical doctors and so-called health experts never come right out and say what normal, average men and women can do to live healthier and longer lives.

"Instead of getting a prescription to follow," she wrote, "you get multiple choices to pick from."

Well, in this book, you will get a "prescription" for healthy longevity. I will tell you, step by step, what actions you should take (and what actions you should avoid) to be able to enjoy a more vital and vibrant life to the age of 90 ... 100 ... perhaps even beyond 100!

No matter how old you are now — whether you're 20 or 50 or 70 — you'll be able to live a longer, fuller, more active life. You'll be able to dance at your great-great-grandson's wedding ... play water polo instead of shuffleboard when you're 90 ... be a snow-skiing granny or grandpa, if that's what you choose ... and still be active and healthy into your second century of life!

The title of this book, *Healthy at 100 — 7 Steps to a Century of Great Health*, is a perfect description of the program you will discover as you read on — a seven-step program that will, if you follow it, add vital decades to your life and enable you to live to be 100 or 105 or even older.

And be assured that this is an easy program to put into practice. You will need to make some lifestyle changes, of course, but these changes will be realistic and gradual — and well worth the effort.

My seven-step program

The seven steps you'll be urged to take in these pages are proven, guaranteed, life-extending actions. They are simple steps. They are sensible. They are easily accomplished. And, as you'll find out as you read on, the effectiveness of this entire program is backed by both medical research and real-world experiences.

- My seven-step program starts with the simple action of taking a personal inventory — making a self-assessment of your current physical condition and any behaviors in your life that threaten your longevity.

- Then, in a logical order, the program gives specific actions you can begin to take immediately to protect your body from the ravages of illness and aging, to strengthen your heart and lungs, to better manage stress in your life, to reduce your body's fat while you add mass and strength to your muscles and skeletal structure, to protect yourself from back problems and injuries, and, finally, to eat tasty and nutritious foods that actually help your body fight diseases including cancer, heart attack, and stroke.

- In addition, I'll give you solid tips on how you can budget your time to make it easier to fit exercise into your daily schedule, and I'll give you specific, illustrated exercise programs for both beginners and intermediates.

- Plus, I'll give you a selection of menus I created that guarantee you to get the proper mix of protein, carbohydrates, and fats in your daily diet.

- I'll also teach you how to take control of your own illnesses — and heal yourself of the most common problems that I see among my patients.

- And, I'll give you a brief outline of the program I have used to help hundreds of my patients "kick" the smoking habit. This section is included because I firmly believe that everyone should quit smoking, and because I know how difficult it can be.

- Finally, I'll fill you in on cutting-edge research that will lead to the most important health-related discoveries of the next decade.

Before you begin ...
The very best way for you to use this book is to start by reading it all the way through so that you get an understanding of my entire seven-step program and exactly what it has to offer you. Then, start again at the beginning, using the book as a guide as you take the specific steps, one by one, to turn back the hands of time and to protect yourself against illness and aging.

The best way to put this program into action is to concentrate on one step at a time. The order in which you incorporate the steps is not important, but be sure to make the step you choose to work on an established part of your life before you move on to the next step.

Go at your own pace

There is no timetable for you to adhere to as you go through the seven steps, other than whatever timetable you set for yourself.

There are two reasons for this:

First, as part of the process, you will have to acquire new habits — the "habit" of moderate exercise and the "habit" of stress management, for example. And experience has shown that it takes anywhere from several months to a year-and-a-half for people to become habituated to new behaviors. There is no way, then, to set a timetable that will be suitable for every man and woman.

Second, the core of my seven-step program is empowerment. This is a program that puts you firmly in control of your own health future. You are the one who will take the actions that will decide how long and in what degree of healthfulness you will live. You are the one who will make the decisions about how fast you want to progress with the individual steps of the program. You have the freedom to put all these steps into practice within a year, if that's your decision. You also have the freedom to take as long as you wish — three years, four, or even five. That freedom gives you the very best chance to successfully put the entire seven-step program into action — the best chance to achieve healthy, vital, and vibrant longevity.

You can do it

Does all this mean that I'm guaranteeing you will comfortably live to be 100?

Of course not. I am guaranteeing, however, that the simple plan you'll find in the pages that follow will lengthen your life and improve your health. I guarantee that if you eat the foods I suggest, if you exercise the way I describe, if you take the vitamins and nutrients I recommend, and, perhaps most importantly, if you learn to make use of and strengthen the unassailable link between your body, your mind, and your spirit, you will live a much fuller, more vibrant, happier, and longer life.

How well and how long you will live depends on your age and physical condition as you begin this program. It depends even more upon the willingness with which you practice these seven steps.

Your life is in your hands

Many of the ideas, principles, and facts you will encounter in this book will be unfamiliar to you, and a few of the things I talk about may be totally new and strange. I ask you to give me the opportunity to share my knowledge with you, remembering that my knowledge has been acquired from two decades of medical practice and from thousands of hours of studying what makes people age and what can keep people from aging.

Along the way, I'll tell you some true life stories about people who are already living longer, healthier, and more active lives as a result of practicing the principles you'll learn here.

And finally, I'll provide you with scientific data and statistical evidence that I believe will make it impossible for you to discount the promise of healthy longevity. In the end, I'm sure you'll be convinced, along with thousands of my patients, that it is possible to minimize the effects of aging, even as you add years or decades to your life.

I hope this book inspires you to improve the life you are currently living. With my program, you can truly change the way you think, feel, and live — and, with a little luck, live to be healthy at 100!

Chapter One

The Promise of Longevity

Shigechiyo Isumi, a Japanese fisherman, lived almost 121 years — and there are thousands of others who have lived to be 100, 110, and even older. Yet, people who live to be 100 are big news in our Western culture. We read about them in our local papers. We hear about them on morning television. We congratulate them and applaud them.

But, why do we applaud? Do we applaud merely because they've lived to be 100? And if so, what does that say about our views on aging and about how long we expect to live ourselves?

It says, I believe, that most of us expect to die long before we reach 100, because we think there is something extraordinary about anybody who lives to be 100. We think this way even though there is no biological reason why we can't all live to be 100 years old or older.

Let me repeat that: *There is no biological reason why we can't — all of us — live to celebrate our 100th birthdays!*

1

Most people don't die of old age

I view any death before age 100 as an early death. How can I possibly say this when most people die long before they reach 100? Easily. Because most people do not die of old age. They die of disease or accident.

As long ago as 1938, a senior pathologist in Great Britain said the same thing when he reported in the medical journal *Lancet* that he had never, in his long professional career, ever performed an autopsy on an individual who died of old age. That all the cadavers he'd had on his table had, instead, died of disease.

More recently, researcher S. J. Olshansky of the University of Chicago's Department of Medicine went high-tech and presented a scenario — based on a computer model — in which the average life expectancy of humans would approach 100.

Olshansky forecast average life expectancy gains that would be realized if high-risk, illness-causing activities (smoking and improper diet, for example) were eliminated, and if the killer diseases cancer, heart disease, and diabetes were removed as causes of mortality. His research, reported in the November 2, 1990 edition of the journal *Science*, showed that, given those circumstances, the average life expectancy for both men and women would leap to about 99.2 years. And his research didn't even take into account the "extra" years that you can gain by taking the additional longevity-extending actions you'll read about in this book!

This, then, is the great news that is at the core of this book. The great news that is at the very heart of the practice of 21st century medicine: *You don't have to die at 80 — or 90 — or even 100!*

You can — more easily than you ever thought you could — remove (or at least mitigate the effects of) high-risk behavior from your life while you protect yourself against killer illnesses. You can even, in many cases, reverse damage that's already been done. In the process, you'll extend your life to the 100 years that are your biological birthright. I say this with full awareness that the current average life expectancy (A.L.E.) in America is 75.4 years (slightly more or slightly less, depending upon sex and race).

Statistics distort the facts

The average age at which Americans die is not in any way a reflection of any individual's personal potential life span. In other words, how long you live doesn't have anything to do with the A.L.E.

To understand more clearly why this is, let's look at a hypothetical culture to see just how erroneous the average life expectancy statistic can be. Let's say this hypothetical culture has a total population of only five individuals. The five individuals die at ages 3, 65, 99, 100, 110. Add these five ages up and the total is 377 years. Divide that 377 years by five and you have an average of about 75 years. Our mini-culture, then, has an average life expectancy of about 75 years, even though three of the five individuals — the majority of the population — lived to be older than 99!

And so it is whenever we look at life expectancies — either in our own culture or in other societies around the world. Some members of every society, because of catastrophic illness or accident, die at an early age. Some die at what we've long mistakenly considered to be about the "normal" age for death. Some live to be 100. And a few approach what most scientists currently say is the true upper limit of the human life span — about 120 years.

Forget about the "average" life span

A human life span of 120 years is not a hypothetical possibility. It is a reality. And the fact that scientists have verified hundreds of such cases indicates — in the simplest terms possible — that most, if not all of us, have the biological capability of living to the ripe old age of 120 years!

So put aside your assumptions about "average" life expectancy. Sure, statistics show that you can expect to live just 75 years. But the newest scientific research is giving you the great news that you are capable of living to be 100, or 110, or even 120. And I'm telling you to forget about dying in your 70s. Learn about the principles and practices of longevity — and then decide for yourself how long you want to live.

First, though, let us look at some of the people who already are living (or have lived) longer and healthier lives.

Who is living longer — and why

Just a few short years ago, the idea that it was possible to lengthen life spans to the century mark and beyond was almost laughable. But now, the idea — or, rather, the promise — that we can live longer, live to 100 years or more, is slowly becoming more widely accepted.

This widening acceptance started with the growing knowledge that many men and women in other cultures live longer and healthier lives than most Americans. This evolving recognition gained strength as scientists started studying, for the first time in any real depth, how people age and what we can do to forestall the effects of aging.

You might remember a series of television commercials that ran several years ago, claiming that eating yogurt was one reason people in a village in the mountains of Afghanistan routinely lived vigorously to 120, 130, even 140 years old. While the yogurt claims may have been exaggerated, the commercial did raise public awareness of the fact that there are pockets of people in the world where men and women routinely live for 90 years or longer.

Dr. Kenneth Pelletier, Ph.D., author of *Longevity: Fulfilling Our Biological Potential*, says that such cases of long life are "not unique ... [and that] instances of healthy longevity of 90 to 120 years have been documented in many other societies since at least the sixth century B.C." To back his claims, Dr. Pelletier cites instances of healthy longevity which have occurred in the Andes and in Pakistan. These instances, he concludes, "are an indication of a biological potential [to live long, healthy lives] inherent to the human species as a whole."

Dr. Pelletier also points out Socrates, the Greek philosopher, who, it is said, lived for 98 years — Heraclitus of Ephesus, another philosopher, who lived for 96 — Pythagoras, the philosopher mathematician, who reportedly died at age 91 — and Michelangelo, who painted the Sistine Chapel and wrote poetry until the time of his death at 89. More recently, Bertrand Russell (yet another philosopher) lived to be 98. Bernard Shaw, the philosopher-dramatist, lived to be 94. Pablo Picasso, the painter, lived to be 92. And playwright George Abbot, at the age of 100, brought a revival of his first hit, "Pal Joey," to Broadway.

Healthy longevity is a scientifically documented reality

To be honest, some reported cases of "healthy longevity" in the Andes mountains of South America, in Soviet Georgia (Afghanistan), and in the mountain valleys of Pakistan were improperly documented, and, therefore, unscientific in their conclusions that it was common for residents in those areas to reach the age of 110 or 120. However, it is now accepted that these enclaves, and a few others around the world, are home to people who, in many instances, do reach the age of 100 in robust good health.

In the U.S., even as interest in the longevity of other cultures is growing, there has been a sharp rise in the number of American men and women who have reached 100. In fact, the number of Americans aged 100 or more is currently estimated by the Census Department at almost 36,000 — double the number of just a decade ago!

An increasing interest in alternative medicine

This awareness of longer life spans among American men and women, and among populations in other parts of the world, has encouraged scientists and physicians in this country to step up research into longevity. These studies, in turn, have led to an increasing interest in what typically is called "non-traditional" or "alternative" forms of medicine.

In 1992, the National Institutes of Health opened its Office of Alternative Medicine. Then, in 1993, press pundit Bill Moyers aired a Public Broadcasting System television series, "Healing and the Mind," that explored the mind-body connection and alternative therapies. This series was overwhelmingly popular with both the public and critics. Even more recently, some of the country's most prestigious scientific and medical journals (including the *New England Journal of Medicine* and the *Journal of the American Society on Aging*) have carried in-depth articles examining the efficacy of non-traditional forms of medicine in promoting longevity.

A new focus on extending life

Scientists are now looking, with open minds, at the lives and habits of aged individuals in the hopes of finding common threads or techniques that would account for their increased longevity.

At the same time, studies conducted in some of the world's top research centers and hospitals already have proved the value of light exercise and weight lifting to promote healthy aging, the ability of antioxidants to ward off or even cure life-threatening disease, and the effectiveness of Asian stress-reduction techniques such as yoga and meditation to promote wellness and slow the aging process.

As a result of this new focus on extending life, the upper limit of the human life span is being pushed back with remarkable speed. Within the next 20 years or so, we're going to stop being surprised when we hear or read about 80-year-olds and 90-year-olds who are leading active lives. We're going to get used to the idea that many more of us than ever before will live to be 100. Newspapers won't even bother sending photographers out to birthday parties for centenarians.

Aging is natural — debility isn't

I'm not saying life will be limitless. Aging is natural and inevitable. Death is natural and inevitable. What is neither natural nor inevitable, however, is feebleness and sickness and pain at 50 or 60, and death at 75.

The fact is that death from "old age" per se is so rare as to be almost unheard of. Instead, Americans are dying from cancer, heart disease, diabetes, or catastrophic accident. And the good news is that you can take actions to (at the very least) drastically reduce your chances of contracting many of the most deadly diseases simply by changing the way you live.

How you can extend your life to 100 — or beyond

In order to live longer then the cultural average — to extend your life beyond the current American A.L.E. of about 75 years — you have to accomplish two basic goals.

The first thing you have to do is "duck bullets" fired in your direction by debilitating and deadly illnesses. You'll be happy to hear that there are many recent studies showing that it is really possible to protect yourself from the life-threatening diseases that most of us simply assume are the necessary baggage of middle and old age. And, though you might think the actions you'll have to take to duck these bullets are complicated or time-consuming, they're not. Avoiding disease and thereby extending your life is a simple matter of making minor changes in the way you live.

The second thing you have to do is take actions that will enable you to slow, stop, or even reverse the aging process. This will make it possible for you — no matter what your age, no matter if you're 30 or 70 — to live not only a longer life, but a healthier, more vibrant, stronger life for all your years.

A huge study of almost 11,500 men and women undertaken by the University of California in Los Angeles found, for example, that if you're a male and you take 500 milligrams of vitamin C daily and get the equivalent of 50 milligrams from food (that's the amount you get in an 8-ounce glass of orange juice), you could add five years to your life. If you're a woman and you take the same amount of vitamin C each day, you can cut your chance of dying from a stroke or heart attack by about 25 percent — and add about an extra year to your life.

These results were seconded by the results of a similar study that examined the health experiences of more than 11,000 men and women over a 10-year period. This study, conducted by researchers from the School of Public Health at the University of California and reported in the prestigious journal *Epidemiology*, found that men in the study whose daily vitamin C intake was equal to two oranges plus a 150-milligram vitamin C pill had a 42 percent lower risk of death from heart disease and a 35 percent lower risk of death from any cause than the population as a whole. Women had a 25 percent lower risk of death from heart disease.

If you were drowning and somebody threw you a life preserver, wouldn't you grab it as quickly as you could and use it to save your life? Of course you would! Well, vitamin C is a life preserver when it comes to heart disease and other killer diseases. Just by taking a daily dose of vitamin C (I'll tell you what my specific recommendation is in Chapter Six), you can "save" your life.

Vitamin E is another lifesaver. In fact, according to a Harvard University study of a group of men and women who took the vitamin daily for more than two years, taking vitamin E regularly can slash your risk of heart attack in half!

I could, if I wished, fill page after page with citations about the efficacy of vitamins in warding off disease. Just the few examples above, however, should provide proof enough that vitamins work. Clearly, they enable us to avoid deadly diseases — including heart attack. Knowing that, you'd be foolish not to take vitamins, right? Yes. Just as foolish as a drowning man who turns his back on a life preserver.

Don't underestimate the benefits of moderate exercise

There are other simple actions you can take to extend your life.

One of the most effective is to begin a program of moderate exercise. I don't mean that you should run 27 miles a day — or work out on an exercise machine for three hours every afternoon. I mean truly moderate exercise.

Let's say you put aside about three hours weekly for walking — enough time to walk nine miles every week. You could, if you wish, go for a walk in a park near your home, walk to the store instead of drive, perhaps even walk to and from work, if that's a possibility for you. It sounds more like recreation than exercise, doesn't it?

And, yet, just this modest amount of exercise can reduce your risk of death by 21 percent. That was the finding of a Harvard University study of 17,000 men that sought to determine the correlation between exercise and longevity.

Research proves that it works

The benefits of moderate exercise can't be overstated. And they've been proved beyond the shadow of a doubt in countless scientific studies. For example, one study sponsored by the University of Utah Medical School showed that a regular program of exercises that most of us consider to be fun (such as bowling, ballroom dancing, gardening, and simple walks around the neighborhood or local mall) reduced the risk of heart attack by 30 percent.

The correlation between moderate exercise and longevity through freedom from disease was also proved by researchers at the Stanford University School of Medicine in Palo Alto, California when they looked at the health habits of 10,269 Harvard University alumni over an eight-year period. They found that moderately active men — men who took part in such sports as jogging, swimming, and running — had a 23 percent lower risk of dying from any cause than men who never worked out.

Of course, most of us have always known that exercise is good for us. Only lately, though, have we discovered that exercise is good for us no matter how old we are. In fact, another long-term study of 10,000 Harvard graduates (conducted by Dr. Ralph Paffenbarger of the University of California at Berkeley) showed that men from 45 to 84 years old who take up moderately vigorous forms of exercise (like tennis, swimming, jogging, or brisk walking) reduce their overall death rates by as much as 29 percent, and have a 41 percent lower risk of coronary artery disease than men who don't exercise.

If you truly want to add years to your life, exercise! It's that simple.

•   A study of 1,960 healthy men aged 40 to 59, conducted by the National University Hospital in Oslo, Norway over a 16-year period, showed that the most physically fit men had half the risk of death of the least fit men.

•   Another study, sponsored by the Institute for Aerobics Research in Dallas, Texas, followed more than 10,000 men and 3,000 women for an average of more than eight years, and found that those in the study who exercised had lower death rates from all causes — as well as lower reported rates of colon cancer, coronary heart disease, hypertension, and stroke.

•   A 32-year study of long-term survival rates of 2,129 Dutch semi-professional and recreational ice-skaters showed rates of death due to all causes at one-quarter below the average rates for men and woman who don't skate.

Each of the studies that I have mentioned so far, conducted by top-notch scientists at some of the world's most famous and best respected research and medical centers, give solid proof that it's possible for average men and women to take simple actions — actions as uncomplicated as walking or jogging and taking vitamins, actions that don't require a huge outlay of time or effort — to make themselves resistant or impervious to disease and aging. These studies take the dream of adding years or even decades to your life out of the realm of make-believe and put it solidly in the realm of scientific certainty.

The importance of the mind-body connection

Other studies present results that may be — at least to the Western mind — even more remarkable. These studies hold forth the promise that the mind can be used to keep the body healthy. Of course, this isn't news to Eastern medical practitioners who come from a culture where it is simply understood that there is an undeniable link between the mind and the body.

Consider, for a moment, the results of a large-scale study of 2,000 older health insurance customers that examined the benefits of stress-reduction techniques, including meditation. In this study, those who followed a daily routine of relaxation exercises had 87 percent fewer instances of heart disease than normal for their age group, 55 percent fewer cancerous tumors, and 87 percent fewer nervous disorders. The mind-body link established in this study — and in others — is only now beginning to be taken seriously by a few medical practitioners in the West.

My own research — and my own practice of techniques that I'll describe in detail in later chapters — has convinced me that one of the best and easiest things you can do to guarantee a long, disease-free life, is to take time each day to relax. In other words, to learn how to manage stress in your life.

You can control your medical future

Based on what we now know, it is obvious that you have the opportunity, as never before, to extend your expected life span. You don't have to resign yourself to falling victim to a life-threatening or life-ending disease as a "natural" part of growing older. You can control your own medical future to an extent that people just a generation ago could not even imagine. You can duck the bullets that kill most people in their 70s, and go on to live to be 100 or even older!

Later in this book, I will describe, in detail, my seven-step program that you can use to stay healthy to 100. I'll tell you exactly what you can do to prolong your healthy life span. But, just to get you started, let me suggest the best thing you can do right now to prolong your life. Something that, though very simple, might well be the single most important action you can take.

The single best thing you can do to live longer

Here's the most powerful longevity secret of all. If you want to live to be 90 or 100 or 110, what you must do, starting now, is think you can. That's right, thinking (and eventually believing) that you will live a long life sets in motion a series of other thoughts and actions that — cumulatively — will help you live longer.

Unless you're 100 already, or just about to celebrate your 100th birthday, that fact in itself should have a powerful impact on your life. If you're 40, you have ahead of you the near-equivalent of what you once believed was a full life — another 60 years or more. If you're 50, you have another 50 years of life to enjoy — maybe even 60 or 70.

Life really can begin at 40

When, in this scenario, does so-called "middle age" begin? Not at 40, surely. Not even at 50. If you're 65, you're not a "senior citizen," no matter how many discount cards you carry. Senior citizens are in their 80s or 90s.

So, if you're 40 and have decided your chosen line of work doesn't make you happy, you have plenty of time to go back to school and prepare yourself for a second career. If you always wanted to learn to play the accordion and never quite had time, now you do. If your spouse passes away when you're 65, you have the option of building a second, long-term relationship.

Accept a new way of thinking

No matter how old you are now, you have a chance to live a longer, healthier, and more vibrant life than at any other time in the history of humanity. But to do this, you must start by believing the evidence that a longer life is yours for the taking. Turn your back on the belief that life is a 75-year journey from youth to old age, from wellness to illness, from vitality to feebleness — and that on this journey you must adhere to some sort of degenerative timetable that gives you just so much healthy time and no more.

Turn your back on the belief, so prevalent in this society, that "productive life" ends when you reach the mandatory retirement age of 65. Or, at the latest, when you blow out the candles on your 75th birthday cake.

Turn your back on the belief that it's normal, even expected, that your body will wear out as you grow older. That by the time you're in your 40s, the old machinery will be starting to show signs of wear and tear. Your knees will creak, your belly sag, your arteries harden, and your bones soften.

And turn your back on the idea that diseases like heart disease and cancer and diabetes and Alzheimer's are an unavoidable part of the aging process.

Why? Because turning your back on these ideas robs them of their strength. Accepting a new way of thinking — namely, that you will live a long and healthy and vibrant life — sets in motion a process that ultimately invests you with the strength you need to make that thought a reality.

I know that it works

I have observed, hundreds of times, the almost magical power of this process at work in my own patients. And scores of my patients have reported back to me how taking this simple step empowered them to begin, immediately, to feel younger, more fit, and more vital. How, in fact, they have become capable of actions they thought were beyond them. How they've become literally stronger — able to lift, and run, and stretch, and work harder and better. How they have even started to look younger to themselves and to those around them.

So, start today by taking this all-important step, knowing that you will immediately gain as a result. Knowing, too, that the results of all the studies I have cited are true: You can take simple steps to add years, maybe even decades, to your life.

In the next chapter, I'll tell you more about ways you can take control of your own body. You'll learn that you can not only live to be 110, but you can live to be a "young" 110 — able to enjoy a life filled with active vitality, sexual energy, and freedom from the pain of those arthritic joints.

Chapter Two

The Essence of Vitality and Well-Being

From the rishis in India, and the gurus of China and Japan, I have learned about the self-healing powers we all have when we live in tune with our natures — or "in balance" as it is called in Ayurveda. And that health, happiness, and vitality is the natural state of our minds and bodies — no matter how long we live.

Imagine being able to jog at full-tilt when you're 70. How about celebrating your 80th birthday by making love with your spouse? Forget shuffleboard. Imagine, instead, water-skiing when you're 90. Imagine bounding out of bed in the morning — no matter what your age — greeting the sun with a yoga stretch, and then being active and without pain for the rest of a full day.

All these things (and more) are possible, if you follow my simple seven-step program for good health.

But first, before you start working on any of the seven steps, you have to learn that what you may think you know about aging is as false as what you thought you knew about the inevitability of death at age 75 before you started reading this book!

Growing older doesn't have to mean growing aged

Just as you now know that it's not true that you have to die at a certain age, you'll learn that growing older does not mean growing into a life of pain and feebleness and decreasing vitality. Just as research and anecdotal evidence point the way to a life span that extends far beyond the average live expectancy of 75 years, they also point the way to a long life filled with vitality, vibrancy, and health.

If you believe that adding years to your life means adding years in which deterioration, pain, and illness are unavoidable — years you're likely to spend in a hospital bed — you might wonder why you'd ever want to live to be 100 or older. If you believe that extending your life for an extra 20 years means no more than giving up wellness in exchange for an extra two decades of painful inactivity, chances are you'd opt for fewer years.

I know that if that were all I could expect from extending my life — namely, the certainty of decay and decline — I'd have to say I wasn't really interested in doing it.

Just living for 100 years isn't enough

I expect to be 126 years old. That's the target age I've set for myself. But I want those "extra" years of mine to be not just a decade or two "tacked on" to the end of my life. I want them to be years that are free from pain and illness and gradual decay. I want them to be filled with happy experiences and growth and activity.

Just plain common sense tells me that many other Americans share my desire for an active, healthy life decades beyond the average life expectancy. There's also statistical evidence that proves that most people don't just want years added to the end of their lives. They want years filled with health and vitality.

One survey, for example, commissioned by *Parade Magazine*, showed that 66 percent of 2,503 respondents said the thing they feared most about growing old was living beyond an age where they could care for themselves and maintain good health.

We know it can be done

Evidence that you can actually slow or even stop the aging process and enjoy additional years of active, vital life far beyond your 60th or 75th birthday is all around us. This evidence has convinced me that there is, in fact, a way for you to add years, maybe even decades, to your life while enjoying good health and well-being that until now you may have associated only with youth.

Consider, for example, Vanacha Temur, whose story was told by Dr. Deepak Chopra, in his book *Ageless Body, Timeless Mind*. Vanacha — a native of Abkhasia, a mountain region in southern Russia — who claimed an age of 110, was visited by a group of American journalists. They found that the old man was spry, alert, and full of life and vitality.

> *"Vanacha's vigor ... was incredible. A man of about five feet with twinkling blue eyes and an elegant white mustache, he was the personification of a kindly and playful grandfather. He credited his slim, wiry body to light eating, horseback riding, farming, and walking in the mountains."*

The old fellow had in his possession a baptismal certificate that showed he was 106 years old. But, he explained, his parents had waited four years to baptize him, while they saved money to pay the priest.

Whether he was 106 or 110, Vanacha, with blood pressure of 120/84, was a remarkable example of healthy longevity. He was not, however, atypical — at least not in his own society. According to Dr. Chopra, a study of Abkhasians aged more than 90 showed that fully 85 percent were mentally healthy and outgoing, only one in 10 had poor eyesight, and only 4 percent had poor hearing.

And then there's Shigechiyo Isumi, the Japanese fisherman who died at 120. According to his doctor, Isumi was healthy and alert until just a few months before his death in 1986.

Such anecdotal evidence that healthy living even at age 100 and beyond is possible has been amassed with increasing regularity in recent years. It has been amassed with enough regularity that we can no longer look at Vanacha and Isumi and others who live healthy lives for 100 years as freaks who somehow beat the odds — as exceptions to the rule that life ends at about age 75.

The difference between chronological age and biological age

To understand how some men and women can actually live to be 100 or even older, it is necessary first to understand and accept that there are two ways to measure age.

1. There is your *chronological age* — your age in the actual number of years you have been alive.
2. There is your *biological age* — your age as expressed by your life signs and by the condition of your body's cells.

Here's a medical fact: Chronological age has little to do with biological age. You've probably made this observation yourself without recognizing how it applies to your own life. For example, do you know a 40-year-old who looks and acts 10 (or even 20) years older? Have you ever met a 70-year-old who looks and acts like 40 or 50? And don't we all know a few ageless and indefatigable "old-timers" who — like the Mississippi River — just keep rolling along, year after year, seeming somehow to grow younger though their chronological ages creep higher and higher?

Your biological age, not your chronological age, determines how long you live and the quality of the life you live, in terms of health and well-being. And, so, it is your biological age that should be of the utmost concern to you.

Now for the bad news/good news

The bad news is that you can do nothing about your chronological age. The good news is that biological aging can be slowed. In fact, in many cases biological aging can be stopped. And in some cases, it can even be reversed! We have overwhelming scientific evidence that this is possible.

Consider, for example, the effects of exercise. Fred Kasch, who, at age 80, is the head of the Exercise Physiology Lab at San Diego State University, has tracked the results of exercise on a group of 12 men for a remarkable 28 years (the longest duration of any such study I know of).

*   One of the men in the study has not gained a pound in 30 years. He has the same blood pressure he had three decades ago, and has the aerobic power (the heart and lung capacity) of a 25-year-old, even though he's a 61-year-old grandfather.
*   Another participant in the long-term study has better aerobic

power (defined by Kasch as the ability of the heart and lungs to deliver oxygen to the body's blood and muscles) at age 75 than he did when he first started exercising at age 47!

I know that you can "grow younger" with my program

What all the scientific research and anecdotal evidence tells me, beyond any doubt, is that you don't have to look forward to growing "old" at 50 and spending the rest of your life dealing with the illness and disease and helplessness that have for generations (at least in America) been associated with the aging process.

This means, for example, that an overweight, out-of-shape, 35-year-old male who smokes and drinks and lives under stress, and who, therefore, has a biological age of 60 or older, can — following the regimen outlined later in this book — quickly reduce his biological age to 50, and then to 45, and then to 40, and even to 35 or 30. The fact is that anyone can "grow younger" just by following my program.

That's right. You have control — in fact, a great deal of control — over just how you age. You don't have to simply sit back and allow your body to deteriorate. You can stop some of the aging processes before they get started. You can inhibit, and even reverse, others that may already have started in your body.

You can control your biological clock

Countless studies dramatically prove that you can turn back the hands of time with exercise, changes in diet, the regular use of vitamins and nutrients, and the use of meditation and other forms of stress reduction.

I've already mentioned that exercise is one of the things you can do if you want to avoid heart attacks and other killing diseases. Research shows that it will help you slow or reverse the biological aging process, as well.

The most remarkable example I've ever come across of the power of simple exercise to reverse the aging process involved 10 residents in a Boston nursing home who were instructed to lift weights three times weekly, for from 10 to 20 minutes each time. Within just eight weeks, these residents — who ranged in age from 86 to 96 — had more than doubled their strength. Even more exciting, two of the 10 had tossed away their canes and were able to walk unassisted for the first time in years. And one man had risen, without help, from a chair that had held him captive! Keep in mind that these were elderly people who were described by Tufts University researcher Maria Fiatarone as "people who are about as sedentary as human beings can possibly be, and almost as old as any human being can be."

Exercise does more than enhance strength

Exercise doesn't just affect your muscles. Part of the process of aging, for example, is a weakening of the immune system — the system that protects the body against common (and uncommon) illnesses. One study, overseen by University of North Carolina exercise physiologist David Nieman, showed that active women in their 70s — women who walk 45 minutes daily — had immune systems just as robust as those of women in their mid-30s.

Another "typical" and seemingly unavoidable symptom of aging is loss of memory and a lessening of the ability to solve problems. Yet, researchers at the University of Kentucky reported that people who do aerobic exercises boost their ability to recall names and perform other mental tasks. These findings mirror those of a University of Maryland study that showed that fit older men and women are better at solving math problems than older people who don't exercise.

Another big problem associated with the aging process — and another element of aging that you probably think is inevitable — is loss of bone mass, or weakening of the body's skeletal structure. This loss of bone mass is one of the leading causes of fractures in the elderly, particularly in women after the onset of menopause. In worst cases, bones are so weakened that just stepping off a high curb can lead to a fracture. And that, in turn, can be disastrous. Each year about 50,000 of our senior citizens die from complications following hip fractures. But, research shows that this doesn't have to happen. For example, in 1993, Everett Smith, director of biogerontology laboratories at the University of Wisconsin's Department of Medicine reported that a group of middle-aged women who did nothing more than hoist five-pound weights once a week for over four years, slowed by 50 percent the loss of bone mass in their arms.

Exercise isn't the only action you can take

There are other actions you can take in addition to exercise to slow or even stop the inexorable sweep of your life-clock's second hand.

Meditation or stress management, as I mentioned earlier, reduces the likelihood that you'll fall victim to a variety of life-shortening diseases, including heart attack and cancer.

Just what can this mean in terms of actual life extension? In terms of adding years to your life span? Well, a study published in 1992 in the *International Journal of Neuroscience* showed that the simple daily use of meditation to reduce stress added as much as 12 years to the lives of older individuals. This means that if your "normal" life span is 75 years, you can extend that to 87 years just by spending a few moments each day meditating.

The list of actions you can take to stay younger longer and add decades to your life goes on.

Particularly exciting is the very latest research into the effects of vitamins and nutrients and healthy eating. A Tufts University study, for example, showed that healthy elderly individuals who took vitamin E supplements significantly improved immune function, and were able to fight off illness as they did when they were younger.

More exciting were results obtained when researchers gave beta-carotene (the substance found naturally in orange and yellow vegetables) to half of 22,000 doctors who took part in the Physician's Health Study, sponsored by Harvard Medical School. After six years, researchers discovered that in a subgroup of 333 men who had signs of coronary disease before entering the study, beta-carotene appeared to mitigate their heart disease. Those receiving the beta-carotene experienced half as many cardiovascular "events" such as heart attack and stroke. In simpler, non-scientific terms, beta-carotene actually reversed the course of the disease in those physicians with heart problems.

Even cancer, probably the most feared of all illnesses — and one that is typically associated with aging — can be held at bay through diet. This was proved when a massive study by the American Institute for Cancer Research showed that people who regularly eat foods high in beta-carotene have a lesser risk of developing cancers of the epithelial tissues such as those lining the mouth, esophagus, stomach, colon, and, especially, the lungs.

I'm convinced!

I'm convinced that it's possible to actually have a biological age (an age measured by your overall health, your heart strength, your lung capacity, your muscle tone and mass, and your bone mass, among other things) far below your actual chronological age.

I'm sure Mavis Lindgren from the little town of Orleans, California, would agree since Mavis — at age 80 — regularly runs 26-mile marathon races.

So would Lucille Thompson of Danville, Illinois. Lucille, at age 88, was troubled by arthritis and decided to take karate lessons in an effort to ease her pain and increase mobility. Two years later, the 4'11" great-grandmother was awarded her black belt and the unlikely nickname "Killer."

Just as it is possible for "Killer" Thompson in the karate dojo and Vanacha in the hills of his native Abkhasia to live healthy lives far longer than most of us ever thought possible, you, too, can enjoy health, vitality, mental sharpness, and freedom from pain far longer than you ever thought you could.

The two basic goals of my program

All the studies I've mentioned, coupled with anecdotal evidence and experiences I had in my years of medical practice, taught me that there are simple steps that can be taken to prolong life by adding healthy, vital, energetic years to anybody's life span. As a result, I developed the program you'll read about in this book as a simple way for my patients — and for you — to accomplish two basic goals:

1. To repair damage done to your body over the years by poor diet, lack of exercise, lack of attention to vitamin and nutrient intake, too much stress, and certain lifestyle choices you may have made.
2. To stop any further damage from occurring.

It's simpler than you might think

At the heart of my program is the knowledge that all the anecdotal evidence and all the scientific studies supporting the thesis that it is possible to live healthy to the age of 100 pointed to only one major culprit in the disease and aging process — a tiny particle known as a "free radical." All the evidence also identified, for me, just a handful of things you have to do to avoid free radical damage

and have a healthier, longer, more vibrant life.
- Exercise.
- Practice daily meditation or some other activity to reduce stress.
- Take daily doses of vitamins E, C, A, and beta-carotene, and the minerals zinc and selenium, and glutathroid, pyenogenal, and other antioxidants.
- Eat a sensible diet.
- Make healthy lifestyle choices.

What you need to know about free radicals

Now, in order for you to be successful with my seven-step program to health at 100, you don't need to know a lot about these things known as "free radicals." All you really need to know is that they have been identified as likely causative agents in some 60 illnesses and conditions (so far!) including heart disease, cancer, cataracts, Alzheimer's disease, rheumatoid arthritis, and diabetes. They even cause wrinkles.

You also need to know that, unfortunately, free radicals are everywhere. Your body is bombarded by free radicals constantly — when you breathe, when you eat and drink water, when you walk, and even when you rest.

Now for the good news.

No, not good news, but great news. News so great that I believe it to be the most important medical discovery since the discoveries of Louis Pasteur and Joseph Lister about the bacteriological causes of infection and contagious disease.

The great news is that there is a way to actually ward off the effects of free radicals — the ultimate aging-agents and life-destroyers — through the use of what scientists know as "antioxidants."

But the great news doesn't stop there, because antioxidants are not a magic substance invented by man. They are not in limited supply, and they're not owned and controlled by a giant corporation willing to sell you a month's supply for $10,000.

What you need to know about antioxidants

Antioxidants are:
- produced naturally in the body (though not in sufficient supply to ward off forever the unceasing attacks by free radicals),

- easily available in the form of vitamins and minerals —
  most notably in vitamins E, C, and A, beta-carotene, and
  the mineral selenium,
- readily available in herbal forms that you can find at most
  health-food stores and,
- found in many foods.

By the simple expedient of supplying your body with antioxidants, you will take one of the most important steps possible toward guaranteeing yourself a long, healthy, vital, and vibrant life.

The impact of lifestyle on health

There's more, though, to staying healthy for 100 years than simply boosting your body's defenses by ingesting antioxidants. What you eat, the type of exercise you do, and even how you think and breathe also play major roles.

The impact of lifestyle choices on health is becoming clearer each day. I could fill pages with examples of how diet, exercise, smoking, and other lifestyle choices can shorten (or lengthen) your life, and either contribute to your health and wellness or lead to debilitating, fatal illness. Just a few samples should suffice:

- The office of the Surgeon General of the Unites States estimates that 90 percent of all lung cancers (about 100,000 new cases per year) are due to smoking.
- High-fat diets have been implicated as culprits, not only in heart disease, but also in colon cancer, prostate cancer, and breast cancer in women.
- The average life expectancy of an alcohol abuser is 15.5 years lower than that of a non-drinker. (In fact, if it weren't for alcohol abuse, the A.L.E. in America would be approximately one full year longer for all men and women.)
- A University of Washington study showed that walking, jogging, or bike-riding for about 45 minutes four times a week increased the ability of older men's bodies to dissolve blood clots, one of the major causes of both heart attacks and strokes. Other studies showed that exercise either reduced risk of or mitigated the effects of osteoporosis (in women), arthritis, and diabetes — and that it boosted immune levels, helped in weight control and stress reduction, and helped older individuals remain mentally sharp.

I'll point you in the right direction

Central to my seven-step program for healthy longevity is, of course, for you to use antioxidants. In conjunction with that, I'll urge you (if there were any meaningful way I could demand it, I would!) to make healthy lifestyle choices, to quit smoking, and to drink only in moderation. Then I'll give you an easy regimen to follow using exercise, diet, and stress reduction to undo damage already done by free radicals, by your lifestyle, and by time itself.

The exact program you follow will be created by you. All I can do is point you in the right direction. You will have to make personal decisions based on your medical history and that of your family, based on your age, weight, and habits, and even on your goals.

It will be up to you, too, to make decisions regarding smoking and drinking alcohol. In the matter of these very personal choices, I do ask you to bear in mind that new research into free radicals and antioxidants confirms what many in the scientific community already know about smoking and alcohol consumption. Namely, that these habits or addictions are killers because they lead to free radical damage. If you choose to drink or smoke, you can mitigate their effects by taking antioxidants and by exercising and eating right. However, I must, in good conscience, warn you that there's no course of antioxidant therapy or treatment I know of that will remove completely (or even to a significant degree) the effects of smoking and drinking.

How long do you want to live?

Before you read any further — before you learn in any more detail about my seven-step program to health at age 100 — I want you to think about how long you want to live and what quality of life you wish to enjoy.

Say you're 30 years old and you want to live to be 120 years old in good health — to spend your last day driving a fancy sports car to pick up a hot date. That's a realizable goal.

Say you're already 70 years old. You want to live as long as you can and, at the same time, you want to undo damage done by decades of smoking and eating too much fat-laden food. That, too, is possible.

Or, perhaps you're like I was not too many years ago. You're in your mid-30s, stressed out from overwork, overweight from too many burgers and fries, out-of-shape and not very happy. And maybe (as I did) you want to add years to your life, feel better, and find a more satisfying way to spend your days. I know it's possible. I did it!

There are two factors to consider

Just how much time you add to your life and what kind of time you enjoy depends on two factors:

1. Your age when you begin to take control of your own health and your own life; and,

2. How far you're willing to go to implement changes in your life that will — no matter if you're 25 or 75 — help keep your body from aging and deteriorating painfully, and will even help your body repair damage that's already been done to it.

Let us look at these two points in a bit more detail.

How old are you now?

How long you live and the quality of life you enjoy depends, to a great extent, on how old or young you are when you begin to take control of your own health. That's just common sense. As much as I'd like to believe that there's a program out there that will guarantee 120 years of life to everybody, that's not the case. A 70-year-old with a history of heart disease who follows my program cannot expect the same results as a 30-year-old athlete who follows the same program.

The 70-year-old will, however, add years to his or her life. Just as important — or even more important — in the process, he or she will feel better and stronger, and will have less pain and more vitality.

Think of the 70-year-old and the 30-year-old as two automobiles. One is a two-year-old sports model with 10,000 miles on its odometer. The other is a classic with 100,000 miles under its belts. The first car is showing just a few signs of wear, while the second is rattling a bit, has bald tires, and needs shocks.

Wouldn't a program of regular preventive maintenance and repair benefit both autos? You bet it would!

But, since the first car started its program in near-new condition, it might be expected to continue running in good shape for 200,000 or even 300,000 miles. The second car's results might not be so striking, but it would be reasonable to expect it to run in much better shape for many more miles than would have been the case without any regular upkeep and maintenance.

The simple fact is that my seven-step program is, in some important ways, exactly like a repair and maintenance program for an automobile.

How far are you willing to go to implement change?

Just as an automobile maintenance program requires the exercise of discipline and effort, so does a program that's guaranteed to keep you alive and healthy longer. Why? Because just as it does a car limited good to burn high-test gasoline if its spark plugs are dirty, so it does your body limited good to eat a diet rich in cancer-fighting nutrients while smoking a non-filtered cigarette.

You are the one who will determine, to a huge extent, how long you will live. You will also determine the very quality of your life — how much freedom from pain you will have, how active and alert you'll be at age 40, 50, 90, and beyond, how much sex you'll be able to enjoy now and later, and how much vitality you'll be able to bring to all your activities. If a longer, healthier life — a life that finds you still healthy at 100 — is your goal, the time to start achieving that goal is today, no matter what your age.

The important thing to remember is that it is never too late or too early to begin putting to work my seven-step program. It can truly add years to your life, whether you are an out-of-shape 65-year-old or a 23-year-old athlete. And you'll start to reap the benefits immediately when you begin using antioxidants and following my recommendations for healthy eating, moderate exercise, and stress reduction.

Anyone can do it

Anyone can change the way they look and feel — even how long they live. Take D. B., a patient who came to my office several years ago after a massive heart attack. She was the picture of bad health — overweight, out-of-shape, tired, stiff, and unhappy.

After talking with me, D. B. made a commitment to follow my seven-step program. And today, at age 50, she is a vibrant, attractive, and slender (5'2", 95-pound) woman. She no longer smokes, eats all she wants (but sensibly), and has a full, active, happy life.

"I feel and look better today, at age 50, than I did 20 years ago," she says. Looking at her, you'd probably agree.

Now, read on to learn exactly how you can set and then achieve your own goal of healthy, pain-free longevity.

Chapter Three

The Making of a 21st Century Physician

I'm sure that by now you have to be wondering just who I am to be telling you how to live to be 126 years old.

It is important for you to realize that my beliefs about living a long, healthy life did not come to me in the controlled environment of a sterile laboratory. Rather, they're the product of my own personal experiences and of my two decades of intellectual detective work as I searched for healthy longevity for myself and for thousands of my patients.

Along the way, I learned that medicine as it is practiced in the Western world certainly does not have all the answers. Continuing my search, I studied the healing arts of the East, and learned that I had to blend both the ancient and the modern systems to achieve my ultimate goal.

As I write this, I am one of a handful of doctors in the United States trained in the 5,000-year-old Indian medical tradition of

Ayurveda. What impresses me about Ayurveda is the fact that it embraces science. Also, unlike some other alternative systems, Ayurveda allows you to work within the Western system of medicine.

So, for example, I can treat my heart patients with both traditional medications and Ayurvedic remedies at the same time. And I do.

Prevention is the key

It took many years of initial study before I came to the realization that *prevention* is the whole point of medicine. I performed thousands of coronary bypass operations and established the only heart surgery program for the state of South Dakota before I recognized that with all my years of education and experience, and with all my high-tech equipment, I wasn't doing what I really should be doing for my patients — or for myself. I wasn't preventing disease and debility.

Based on that understanding, and everything that I eventually learned from my ongoing studies of both Eastern and Western medicine, I discovered a revolutionary new form of medicine that has the promise to keep people alive and healthy until they are well past 100 years old.

The beginnings of a life-long commitment

When I was growing up on the streets of New Jersey, I had no concept of the man I would become. But I realize now that my heart-felt attitudes about life and living began there.

I have never forgotten, for example, one spring day when I was 13, playing baseball in a Newark park. A police car pulled up with a friend of mine named "Crazy Benny" in the back seat. Benny had been brutally beaten and was being escorted around the neighborhood so he could identify the boys who had attacked him.

I don't recall if Benny's attackers were ever caught. But I do remember that Benny died just a few days later.

At that moment, and in unforgettable terms, I learned of the frailty of human life. And I learned, even at that young age, that life is a precious gift and that every day should be filled with as much positive action and thought and feeling as possible.

I started on a degree in biology

All I really wanted to do when I was growing up was play sports.

Actually, my passion for football is what started me on my academic career. I had visions of myself as a college football star — maybe even a pro. With that in mind, I headed for Boston College.

I majored in biology, with neither any real career plans nor any idea of how I could put a biology degree to good use. I also tried to win a walk-on spot on the Boston College football team. At the end of a year, most of which I spent being mercilessly pummeled by 260-pound linemen, I realized I wasn't going to play varsity ball at the college level and that, if I wanted to graduate, I'd better concentrate on academics and not athletics.

At this point, I had my sights set on a Ph.D. in biology (I hadn't yet even thought about a career in medicine), but I couldn't afford graduate school. So, in my senior year, I figured I would leave school and go into the Army so I could save up some money and use the G.I. Bill to fund the rest of my education.

That's when a biochemistry professor talked me into applying, instead, for a graduate school fellowship. At the time, I didn't even know what a fellowship was, but I took a chance and applied for biology fellowships to Seton Hall University, Rutgers University, and Fordham University. I was accepted by all three, but decided to accept Seton Hall's offer because of its proximity to my family, and because Seton Hall offered me not only free education but also a teaching assistantship that paid me enough to get by with a few dollars left over.

This is when I learned to love research. I published four articles in scientific journals, was awarded a fellowship from the National Institutes of Health, finished tops in my class, and was invited to transfer to the medical school.

I took the opportunity to go to medical school

Reasoning that I could earn my doctorate in biology along with an M.D. and then go on to enjoy a rewarding and challenging life as a researcher and teacher, I transferred to Seton Hall's medical school in a Ph.D./M.D. program.

The balance of my education can only be described as a steady, uphill grind. During my second year at Seton Hall, the four individuals responsible for overseeing my progress through the Ph.D. program left to pursue their own careers. So, suddenly, as I reached the half-way point in my Ph.D. program, I found myself without a committee under which to continue my work. I had no choice but to transfer to a new medical school, even though I'd finished about 75 percent of the research work needed for my advanced degree. I chose the University of Missouri in Columbia.

From the moment I entered the clinical realm of medicine in my junior year, I fell in love with the pursuit of medical knowledge. At that point, I chose to concentrate fully on medicine instead of splitting myself between medicine and biology. This is a decision I've never regretted. To this day, I have not found anything more fulfilling than being able to help people feel better and healthier and more vibrantly alive.

The pressure started to build

Medical school is, however (as any doctor can tell you), a pressure cooker with the heat turned up as high as possible. My personal pressures increased when I got married and, within a year, started a family. True to my upbringing — practicing the work-ethic I learned from my father — I knew I could cope if I just worked harder and worked more hours. And, so, I worked nights as a security guard, went to medical school, and then spent any remaining hours doing my research.

It was at this time that I fell victim to the fallacy that the human body can get by on a mere three hours of sleep a day. The only thing that kept me going during this period was that I was in such good physical condition — the result of my years as an athlete.

Finally, I graduated with honors from the University of Missouri Medical School. And there I was, an Irish-Italian kid from the streets — the first one in my family to get past high school — with a degree in medicine.

Coping with growing demands

After completing medical school, I started surgical training at the University of Michigan. By this time, our second child was born, I had accumulated more than $60,000 in educational debt, and the U. of M. was paying me the princely sum of $5,900 a year as a surgical intern. I moved through my residency, working longer and longer hours.

To give you an idea of just how demanding medical training is, during my internship I was on call each and every night for seven months of my year-long stint on rotation in urology, orthopedic surgery, general surgery, and the emergency room. At one point during this period, one of my children actually told his playmates that I was dead simply because he had not seen me during an entire three-month period.

The mix of intense competition to get the best residency position possible, constant lack of sleep, unremitting scrutiny from professors of medicine and surgery, and near back-breaking financial worries often creates serious problems for aspiring physicians. These pressures, at their worst, can result in depression (even suicide), drug and alcohol dependency (even addiction), and mistakes in judgment that can cost patient lives. They can also lead to family problems and divorce, which, in fact, is where they led in my case.

Important lessons learned along the way

Fortunately, for me, my love for the practice of medicine was (and is) so great that I managed to make it through. Along the way, I learned valuable lessons about life and about myself. I experienced the wonder of being able to save lives. At the same time, I came to realize that my ability to save lives depends on the opportunities and talents that were given to me by God. Most important, I maintained my awareness of the frailty of human life — my own and that of my patients — that I had learned from "Crazy Benny." I was not a superman. Yet, I knew that I had chosen a profession that placed tremendous physical and emotional demands on me.

In 1973, as my marriage was coming to an end and I was becoming a single parent with three children to raise, this understanding that my own health could be endangered by my career forced me to begin making a few changes in the way I lived my life. As a result, I discovered that it was okay for me to read a book that had nothing to do with medicine, that it was okay to sleep for eight hours at night — and that I could do both if I forced myself to free up time away from work. I even started listening to music again, just for pleasure.

Still, this was a difficult time as I struggled to complete my residency and raise my children. I was overwhelmed by my responsibilities — and I wasn't paying nearly enough attention to my own well-being.

At last!

Finally, in 1975, I completed my training at the University of Michigan. From Michigan I moved to Sioux Falls, South Dakota, where I spent the next seven years building a career. This was the most rewarding period of my early career. I was the first board-certified cardiac surgeon in the state, starting the state's first open-heart surgery program while I taught classes at the University of South Dakota Medical School, then in its infancy.

An experience that changed my life

One day, in the operating room, I had a revelation that changed my life — professionally and personally.

I was preparing to replace a valve in a patient's heart. I looked down on that table, and saw this poor guy with his chest sawed open — and realized that this was not the answer.

He was like just about every other patient who came across my table — overweight and overworked, a smoker, somewhere between 45 and 55 years old. I knew that after surgery, chances are he would go back home, and go right back to doing what it was that made him sick in the first place.

Because that's what most of my patients did. Many of them wound up in my operating room two and three times — to undergo the same harrowing procedures. Only each time, the risks were much higher.

I realized at that moment that I was doing little or nothing to make my patients healthy — I was simply prolonging their deaths. I knew that I had to find a better way to help them.

I took a good look at myself first

At the same time, I realized that I was headed down the same road as my patients. Driven to succeed, I was working more than 100 hours a week, smoking a pack and a half of cigarettes a day, and chowing down on 12-ounce steaks for dinner. The only exercise I got was picking up a scalpel.

While my practice was growing, so was my body. I weighed 225 pounds. My life was, to a large extent, out of control. I knew that if I continued the way I was going, someday soon I'd be the one on the table with my chest open. And when I learned that the average thoracic surgeon died between the ages of 54 and 56, it looked like I was right on track to becoming no more than another medical statistic.

I started to get back in shape

A friend of mine, Dr. Larry Seidenstein, encouraged me to exercise — both as a way to lose weight and to reduce job-related stress. At his urging, I entered a three-mile race, realizing that I was about to make my first real attempt at purely physical activity since leaving college.

One week before the race, I thought I'd warm up by running a mile. Imagine my surprise (remember, I had been an athlete) when I discovered that it was all I could do to run about 20 yards, then walk about 50 yards, then run, then walk, just so I could make it through the mile.

The following week, I did manage to pant my way through the three-mile race. But afterwards, I felt so weak that I could barely drive the 70 miles back home. Disgusted with myself, I proclaimed for all to hear, "I'll never be unfit again!" And I meant it.

I began jogging on a regular basis, and the improvements came quickly. My weight dropped to 165 pounds, and within six months I ran in my first marathon — a distance of 26.2 miles — along with my 63-year-old father. My father, by the way, had just started running in his 60s. Not only that, but he finished the marathon about six minutes before me, and was feeling invigorated as he crossed the finish line. It was all I could do to collapse across the line. But I didn't give up, and eventually — in 1984 — I fulfilled one of my dreams by going to Hawaii and competing in the Ironman Triathlon (a 2.4 mile swim, followed by a 112-mile bike ride and a 26.2 mile run).

My own experience inspired me

When I was in medical school, I spent only about four hours studying the effect of nutrition on the body. And even less time studying the effect of exercise and stress management. These factors were simply not considered to be important for good health. However, as I continued with my own quest for fitness, I learned just how critical these factors are.

I learned more and more about the benefits of a high-fiber, low-fat diet, finally becoming an ovo-lacto vegetarian in 1977. I began a regular program of stress management, and as I continued to exercise and change the bad habits I had developed, I felt better and better.

Inspired by my personal success, I began a cardiac rehabilitation program to teach patients with heart disease what I had learned about the overwhelming benefits of physical activity, nutrition, and stress management. In all my years of surgically replacing blood vessels in damaged hearts, I'd never taught my patients to change themselves. And now, I wanted patients to know that surgery was a waste of time if it wasn't accompanied by lifestyle changes.

In 1977, this was progressive — even radical — thinking.

Now, of course, we know that exercise, nutrition, and stress management (the linchpins of my seven-step program for health at 100) are not adjuncts to surgery at all. They are, instead, the treatment of choice for most cases of coronary artery disease. (They're also the tools you can use to extend your life and stay healthy while you're doing it.)

My career took off in a new direction

Over the course of the next four years, it became increasingly obvious to me that the future of medicine and health care in the United States was prevention — not cure. That my duty as a doctor was to teach patients how to avoid surgery and medication — to teach them how to take control of their lives by making intelligent lifestyle changes.

At this time in my life, I found a guide I sorely needed in Dr. George Sheehan, a cardiologist who, at age 50, discovered that he could run his way back into good physical condition. Dr. Sheehan became a vociferous proponent of running for exercise. He was the "guru of all runners" at a time when most physicians did not stress the benefits of physical exercise at all. And he gave me help and encouragement as I explored new ground, learning lessons that were to have a profound impact on me and on the thousands of patients I would treat in the following 15 years.

I was also fortunate to spend time with Dr. Kenneth Cooper, author of *The Aerobics Way*, one of the original texts on the value of exercise, and founder of the aerobics institute bearing his name in Texas. The Cooper Institute has given us much valuable information about the benefits of exercise, and Dr. Cooper, through his writings and teachings, has started literally millions of people around the world on the road to good health.

Thanks to the influence of Cooper and Sheehan, and the lessons that I was beginning to learn about the healing properties of the mind-body connection that is taught in the East, I was able to look beyond what had been my horizons for all those years and to look at my career in an entirely new way. I saw, with amazing clarity, the potential of an exciting new approach to medicine that would make it possible not only to reverse coronary artery disease and other diseases — but to prevent them from ever occurring.

I had discovered a new type of medicine

I had always said that surgery was a young man's career and that when I reached age 45 I would quit and seek a new life. Now, at age 39, I had discovered the beginnings of a new type of medicine that I truly believed in and loved practicing.

So, I took a leave of absence from my practice to teach patients about nutrition, and the proper use of supplements, exercise, and meditation. By 1981, I decided to leave the surgical suite forever and never go back to operating.

My new medical career

My new medical career began in earnest when I was recruited to begin rehabilitation programs for a large hospital district in South Florida. From this project, I made a move into nonsurgical sports medicine, and expanded my practice to include what I call wellness-oriented or preventive sports medicine. My current practice in Boca Raton deals with everything from the practice of Ayurvedic medicine to cardiac rehabilitation, to stress management, to counseling patients on taking control of all aspects of their lives.

I have put hundreds of patients through my cardiac rehabilitation program (logging more than 30,000 patient-hours) and have accumulated overwhelming evidence through this program that when a patient begins regular exercise, his or her physical health improves within months, and the risk of heart disease is reduced by at least half.

But the most important and rewarding part of my practice has been to teach that with fitness, good nutrition, vitamin and mineral supplements, and meditation, we can control, and even prevent the illnesses that lead to debilitation.

Let me show you what I mean ...

A 56-year-old nurse entered my program a few years ago. Her

history was very simple. She had suffered from high blood pressure for 20 years, weighed 185 pounds, and had 35 percent body fat.

She was taking three medications to control her blood pressure. She was taking another medication to control a case of diabetes that was brought on by the blood pressure medications. And she was taking a fifth medication for heart failure.

Three months after entering my program, she was down to 160 pounds. She no longer had to take the diabetes and heart failure pills. She was able to drop two of the blood pressure prescriptions and reduce the dose on the third to half of what she'd been taking.

After 20 years of diabetes, she had it controlled within three months by using what I taught her about alternatives to drug therapy.

I learn more every day
More recently, I have learned that neutralizing free radicals with antioxidants can actually slow the aging process — bring it to a screeching halt or even reverse it — so that there's no longer the need to spend the last years of our lives with chronic illness and steady physical decline.

All told, it has taken me almost 20 years to learn the lessons I have learned. I've learned that while my career is of major importance to me, I can't live my whole life through my work. To be sure, my job as a teacher and healer — like all serious endeavors — requires tremendous dedication and a great deal of time. Yet, I can't let my career become the be-all and the end-all of my life.

To live a long, healthy, vital, and contented life, I must take the time to care for myself. I must stay in control of my life, and not let my life control me. I must — to use the motto I coined years ago when I first started teaching about the benefits of nutrition and exercise — "keep my miles high and my calories low." That means, in simple terms, that I must exercise on a regular basis and restrict my fat intake to less than 20 grams daily.

Knowing what I know about free radicals, I must eat properly and take dietary supplements to counteract and reverse the effect they have on disease and aging.

In addition, I must recognize the link between a healthy body and a healthy mind, and practice stress reduction techniques to manage the pressures in my life. Essentially, I must learn how to relax and have fun as I did when I was a boy.

Finally, I have to accept the responsibility for my own health and physical well-being.

Learn from my experience

To live a long, healthy life, you must do the same. Does this mean you have to become a vegetarian and run in an Ironman Triathlon, or even jog every day, as I have done? No! Not at all! It means that you must find your own way to exercise, and your own healthy diet and lifestyle.

Just as I changed and overcame obstacles placed in my path — so can you. Just as I moved myself to a place where a life of good health for 126 years is possible — you can do the same.

In the chapters that follow, I will teach you simple techniques that you can use to change your life.

As a former hard-driving, overweight, sedentary smoker who used these same techniques to find a life of health and vitality and happiness, I can testify from personal experience that they really work. And that it's easy to get from there to here.

So   if you're ready   now is the time to follow me and start your journey toward healthy longevity.

Chapter Four

The Commitment to Change

I'm going to open a door for you. On the other side of that door, you'll find all the tools you'll need to lead a healthy and vital life for 100 years or even longer. Tools that will enable you to change your whole life and the way you live it — to make your heart, lungs, and muscles stronger, to strip fat from your body and replace it with muscle, to free yourself from back pain, to manage stress in your life, and to enjoy a vibrant sex life no matter what your age.

You'll also find the tools you need to actually ward off the effects of aging, protect yourself against heart attack, stroke, cancer, and other illnesses — and even reverse many disease processes.

But right now — before I open that door to you — I want you to make a simple, yet unconditional, commitment.

I want you to make a contract with yourself to do your best to exercise according to my "Rule of 3s" — to take part in some sort of aerobic exercise or sport for 30 to 60 minutes, three times a week, for three months.

That's all.

Not to become a world-class athlete. Not to train yourself to run a five-minute or six-minute mile. But to do your best, your very best, to do some sort of aerobic exercise for 30 to 60 minutes, every other day, for a three-month period.

The exercise you choose can be as simple as taking a walk in the park. Or you can jog or work out on a rowing machine. Do whatever you enjoy and whatever is comfortable.

Sound easy?

It is.

But, without this commitment, you may as well put down this book right now. Because your sense of responsibility is the foundation upon which all your future gains will be built. Without this commitment, success will be less likely.

The importance of commitment

My own experience of changing from an overweight, over-worked, out-of-shape wreck into a healthy, happy man capable of competing in triathlons taught me just how important commitment is. It also taught me that it's necessary to take one step at a time to put that commitment to work.

If you remember, I did not change overnight. My change started when — urged by a friend to enter a three-mile race — I realized how terribly out-of-shape I was, and I decided to begin running. Other changes followed. I started a program of weight training to go along with aerobic exercise. I made changes in my diet that included my decision to become an ovo-lacto vegetarian. I began practicing meditation and stress-reduction techniques. And, most recently, I began using dietary supplements to give my body added protection against disease and aging.

My own commitment to change was easy once I realized that I was putting my life in jeopardy by not changing. I first had to admit that I'd lost control over my own health. Then I was able to accept the fact that, unless I took action, I was headed for serious health problems and an early death.

I have to assume that you already accept the idea that you need to make some changes in your life, or you wouldn't have read this far in a book that's all about change. And I'm hoping that you accept — in your gut, not just in your mind — the fact that you are the one who is responsible for these changes. Because it's all up to you. Unless you take action — nothing will happen.

Don't look back on your life with regret

One of the heirs to the J. Paul Getty fortune said, when he was in his 80s and close to death, that he regretted that he had spent his whole life making money. He was sad, he said, that he'd never taken the time to use his money in any meaningful way. He'd never traveled for the fun of it — had never taken the time to learn anything other than what he needed for business. He said he was terrified, as his death approached, that his last words were going to be, "I wish I had taken the time to ...."

The same basic sentiments are expressed by an anonymous poet who wrote:

> *If I had my life to live over, I would relax more*
> *I wouldn't take so many things so seriously*
> *I would take more chances*
> *I would climb more mountains*
> *I would swim more rivers*
> *I would ride more merry-go-rounds*
> *I would pick more daisies*
> *The next time, I'd start barefoot earlier in the*
> *spring and stay that way later in the fall*
> *I would not make such good grades in school*
> *unless I really wanted to*
> *I would relax more.*

I find the words of both the anonymous poet and the Getty heir to be profoundly moving. It is bad enough that they both speak with such sorrow about opportunities lost. What is worse, at least in my mind, is that their words indicate an acceptance of the status quo. They have simply given up and accepted the idea that they can't change the course of their lives.

Oh, I know you can't relive your past and make it different any more than I can recapture the time I lost when my whole life was centered around my career. You can, though, learn from your past.

You can look back at your life, take stock of what you've done, and say to yourself, "Okay, I've made mistakes. I haven't taken charge of my own life. I haven't stopped to smell the roses. I haven't taken care of myself. But now I'm going to change. I'm going to be the master of my own fate. I'm going to do things differently!"

Close the door on the past

I ask you — urge you — to close the door on your past the way you'd close the door on a room you never want to see again. You really can't do anything about what you did (or didn't do) yesterday. Then open the door to the future and start living your new life — a life in which your past mistakes and shortcomings play no role except to serve as lessons on what not to do.

Immediately after I ran in my first three-mile race, I decided to shut the door on my past and move on to a new, healthier life. I didn't want to find myself 80 years old and in poor health, bemoaning the fact that I hadn't climbed any mountains or taken the time to walk barefoot in the surf. To make sure that I didn't end up like the anonymous poet, I immediately opened the door to a new way of life.

Was it easy?

In all honesty, there were times when it was difficult. Times when it was tough to exercise at the end of a long day — when it was hard to make the time to prepare a proper meal instead of falling back on pre-packaged convenience foods. But it was easier than I thought it was going to be.

Just get started

My experience tells me that you, too, will find change easier than you imagine once you finally get started. And you get started by making the commitment I asked you to make at the beginning of this chapter. By making a contract with yourself to do some sort of aerobic exercise for 30 to 60 minutes, three times a week, for three months. When you make this commitment, you will be accomplishing two major goals.

1. You will be admitting you need to change.
2. You will be taking the all-important first step to realizing that change.

If, at first, you're unable to live up to your contract — if, for example, you exercise for just two weeks and then give up — that's okay. You can start over again, at any time, so long as the end result is three consecutive months of aerobic exercise. The purpose of this commitment is to enable you to see the benefits that accrue from making even a minor, healthy lifestyle change.

Why this particular commitment?

We're all the products of an impatient society. A society in which we've been taught to expect instant gratification. And aerobic exercise is the fastest and simplest way I know of for you to begin to change yourself. I know — I guarantee — that almost as soon as you start to exercise to lower your body fat, you'll feel better. And when you look in the mirror — you'll see results!

While there are many kinds of aerobic exercise, at this point you should consider putting walking or jogging at the top of your list. I recommend these activities in the beginning, because you can do them without joining a gym or a health club, and without spending a lot of money on equipment. These are also activities that most people find enjoyable.

Actually, a brisk walk is not only the easiest way to start a program of aerobic exercise, it's also one of the most efficient. Many people have reported that walking — around the neighborhood or around an air-conditioned mall — led to changes in physical condition and feelings of health and well-being that exceeded their wildest expectations.

Later, perhaps, you'll decide to buy an exercise machine — a rowing machine, a stationary bike, or even one of the "Nordic Track" type machines — but for now, choose an activity that doesn't involve a big expense.

You can find the time

You may think you can't possibly fit three exercise sessions each week into your already overcrowded, busy schedule. But you can. I have many patients who are busy executives or single parents. Inevitably, the first time I talk to them about exercising three times a week for 30 minutes or more, they swear they can't possibly fit exercise into their busy schedules. But once we look carefully at the way they spend their time, we're able to fit in the exercise.

The first step is to make sure you pick an activity you like. I know from my own experience and from my work with my patients that you will find a way to make the time to do something pleasurable. In fact, I know that once you start a form of exercise you truly enjoy, you'll quickly reach a point where you wouldn't miss one of your thrice-weekly sessions for anything.

Next, sit down with a pad of paper and a pen and write out a schedule showing your daily activities over the course of a typical week. Then examine your schedule and see what you can do to free up some time.

- Maybe you watch the morning news for 30 minutes before you leave for work, and then the evening news for 60 minutes after you return home. Cut out one or the other three times a week, and exercise instead.
- Perhaps you take an hour for lunch every day. Take a short lunch every other day, and spend the time you save walking or jogging.
- Be creative. Take a quick shower instead of a long, lazy tub bath. Skip a situation comedy that you usually watch — or tape it and watch it another time. Consider cutting back on your work hours.

Schedule your exercise sessions the same way you schedule appointments or meetings. What you're doing here, after all, is finding the time to add healthy years to your life.

By shifting activities, I found the time to run from six to 10 miles, five times a week, when I was working 20-hour days as a cardiac surgeon. To be sure, it took some ingenuity on my part. For example, I did paper work on my coffee breaks, and I read in the bathtub.

I'm sure you have the same kind of ingenuity. Even if you work a back-breaking 12 hours a day, seven days a week, and sleep for eight hours a day, you still have four hours a day (28 hours a week) for other activities. Out of that 28 hours, you only need a maximum of three hours a week for your aerobic exercise schedule. If you're serious about your health, you'll do what you have to do and find that time.

Seven more ways to find extra time

Here are some more ways you can find the time you need to

exercise:

1. Prioritize, prioritize, prioritize. When you analyze your daily or weekly schedule, you'll find small sacrifices you can make for the sake of exercise. Perhaps you can go to sleep a little earlier at night, so you can wake up a little earlier in the morning. Or perhaps you can take a commuter train instead of driving your car, so you can work on your way to and from the office.
2. Schedule real "power lunches" — two-hour breaks away from the office when you can both eat lunch and exercise.
3. Consider exercising before you go home from work — as a regular extension of your work day. You may find it easier and more efficient to exercise before you go home to shower, eat dinner, and relax.
4. Leave your car in the driveway and walk or ride a bike to the store when you run errands — or to work if you live close enough. I rode a bike to and from my office, about 10 miles a day, five days a week, when I trained for my first Ironman Triathlon. When I drive to work now, I pass one fellow who walks to work every day. In the last eight weeks, I've seen this man's body go through some amazing changes — I've literally seen pounds melt off his frame.
5. Try to think like a child who is figuring out a way to make time for play. Children always find a way to do the things that are important to them. You need to do the same.
6. When you take public transportation, get on and off at a stop that's a little farther away, and walk the extra distance.
7. You don't need a "cool-down" day between aerobic sessions, so you can exercise two days in a row on the weekend. Then you'll only have to find one more hour for exercise during your busy work week.

Take one step at a time

Once you've made your commitment to exercise for at least 30 minutes a day, three times a week, for three months, be wary of taking on any more — at least in the beginning. In my experience, many men and women who are serious about making important health changes can become almost compulsive. They want to change everything immediately. If you try to do this, you're bound to fail — particularly if you haven't paid any attention to your health for years.

I am not saying that you shouldn't be excited at the prospect of good health. I hope that you're "chomping at the bit," ready to leap into this program and proceed at top speed. However, in the beginning, it is important to take one thing at a time. Don't try to change everything all at once.

Don't give in to negative thoughts

Don't let yourself be trapped into failure by believing that you can't succeed.

- No matter how old you are, you're not too old to be physically active. There's no such thing as being too old to begin some sort of exercise program.
- You're not doomed by heredity to be overweight. No one has to be overweight unless he or she chooses to be overweight.
- There's no reason for your life to be out of control. But recognize that you are the only one who can take charge. When you accept that responsibility and begin to change the areas in your life that need change, you'll be well on your way to a happier, healthier, and ultimately longer life.

Why do I say "happier?"

Because I know from experience that as soon as you get started on a more physically active lifestyle, you'll be better able to cope with the stresses of everyday life. Your self-esteem will be enhanced. You'll be more content in your work. You'll be more creative and productive. As a result of all this, you'll be more satisfied and happy with your life as a whole.

Actions to Take

• Recognize that you need to make some changes if you are to achieve your goal of living a longer, healthier life.

• Make a commitment to begin my program by exercising for 30 to 60 minutes, three times a week, for three months.

• Make an exercise schedule. Prioritize, reorganize, sacrifice if you need to — but make sure you have specific blocks of time set aside for exercise.

Chapter Five

Step 1:
The 20 Questions
That Could Save Your Life

The rishis of India say, "If you want to know the state of your mind yesterday, look at your body today. If you want to know how your body will look in the future, evaluate your mind today." So, before you can take action to guarantee yourself healthy longevity, you must determine exactly where you stand, today, right now, in terms of your health. More specifically, you must determine exactly where you stand in terms of *risks* to your health. Then, you can begin removing, one by one, the major factors that could unnecessarily shorten your life.

If you were about to purchase a business, one of the first things you'd do is take an inventory. You'd look at the company's books, study its history, search out its weaknesses so you could build them up, and determine its strengths so you could capitalize on them. You'd want to know as much as you could about every aspect of the business's health before you put any of your capital at risk.

In fact, you'd follow pretty much the same procedure if you were about to buy a used car, ask your boss for a long-overdue salary increase, or embark on a cross-country motor trip. Because the inventory-taking process is a necessary step for success in virtually any endeavor.

In recent years, health inventories (officially known as health-risk assessments) have become routine for employees of many major U.S. corporations. They're routine because it's been proven, over time, that they promote wellness and save companies millions of dollars in health-care costs.

Just as assessing your health makes sense, it also makes sense that an assessment or health inventory, all by itself, is worthless unless you take action to correct or mitigate any problem areas you find. In other words, the assessment itself won't improve your health or add years to your life unless it results in changes in your health-related, longevity-related activities and behaviors.

While you can, if you wish, have a health-risk assessment administered by your physician (for a fee of $100 or so), it's not necessary. You can easily perform your own assessment by answering the few simple questions listed on the following pages. This assessment is one I developed over the years to help my patients discover any health dangers or deficiencies they need to address. It is the perfect way for you to start my program for healthy longevity.

Your Health-Risk Self Assessment

In the next few pages, I'll ask you a series of questions, first about your family history, then about your lifestyle, then about your general cardiovascular health. In each instance, circle your answer and enter the number of points indicated for that answer, either in the spaces provided or on a separate sheet of paper. When you're done with the assessment, I'll help you evaluate your answers and I'll make some recommendations about courses of action you can take to reduce your own risk.

Now, the questions:

Section 1 — Your Family History

Why look at family history? Because heredity is such an important risk factor in many diseases that lead to death.

Does this mean that if your father died of a heart attack or if your mother died from colon cancer that you'll necessarily die the same way?

No! It does, however, mean that you have an increased risk of heart attack or cancer of the colon. And, knowing that you are at increased risk, you should take specific steps (we'll talk about them at length later) to mitigate or remove, as much as possible, that risk from your life.

  a. How many people in your immediate family (grandparents, parents, aunts, uncles, brothers, sisters) have had a heart attack?

None	=	0 points
1 or 2	=	1 point
3 or more	=	2 points

                                   Your Score_____

  b. How many people in your family have had diabetes?

None	=	0 points
1 or 2	=	1 point
3 or more	=	2 points

                                   Your Score_____

  c. How many people in your family have had cancer?

None	=	0 points
1 or 2	=	1 point
3 or more	=	2 points

                                   Your Score_____

YOUR TOTAL FOR SECTION 1_____

Section 2 — Your Lifestyle
    The importance of assessing your lifestyle can't be overstated
in determining just how much risk you face and deciding what actions you should take to minimize that risk.
    Keep in mind that a behavior like smoking or a sedentary
lifestyle by itself has a negative effect on your health. At the same
time, these damaging factors, when coupled with a family history
of certain diseases, can be downright deadly.

a. Do you smoke?
    Never   =   0 points
    Cigar or Pipe   =   1 point
    Cigarettes:
        None for 8 years+   =   0 points
        None for 3 to 7 years   =   1 point
        Less than 1/2 pack/day   =   4 points
        1/2 to 1 pack/day   =   6 points
        More than 1 pack/day   =   8 points
                                     Your Score_____

b. How's your weight? Score yourself on *either* b-1 *or* b-2 —
not both. If you know your percentage of body fat, it's preferable
to score yourself on b-1, rather than on weight.

    b-1. What's your percentage of body fat? (For more informa-
    tion on determining your body fat percentage, see Chapter
    Eleven.)

        Male: Greater than 25%   =   2 points
                 25% or less   =   0 points

        Female: Greater than 30%   =   2 points
                 30% or less   =   0 points
                                     Your score _____

    b-2. Are you overweight? (If you don't know your body
    fat percentage, determine if you are overweight by using
    one of the formulas on the following page, which provide
    an ideal weight for a healthy individual.)

For a man: Multiply your height in inches times 2, then add 10 to find your ideal weight. For example, the ideal weight for a 6-foot man would be 154 pounds: 72 inches x 2 + 10 = 154.
For a woman: Multiply your height in inches times 2, then subtract 10 to find your ideal weight. For example, the ideal weight for a 5'4" woman would be 118 pounds: 64 inches x 2 - 10 = 118.

Less than 15 lbs. over	= 0 points
15 to 30 lbs. over	= 1 point
More than 30 lbs. over	= 2 points
	Your Score_____

c. What's your stress level?

Low (always happy, giving, and calm) =	0 points
Moderate (angry or worried at times) =	2 points
High (mind constantly active, either with business or family worries or projects) =	4 points
	Your Score_____

d. How active are you?

Very active (aerobic exercise 3 or more times weekly) =	0 points
Moderately active (aerobic exercise 2 times weekly) =	1 point
Slightly active (exercise once weekly, non-aerobic) =	2 points
Sedentary =	4 points
	Your Score_____

e. How's your diet?
(1) How much water do you drink each day?

8 to 10 glasses	=	0 points
5 to 7 glasses	=	1 point
4 glasses	=	2 points
Less than 4 glasses	=	4 points
	Subscore_____	

(2) How many whole fruits do you eat each day?
   At least 3   =   0 points
   Less than 3   =   4 points
        *Subscore*_____

(3) How many cooked vegetables do you eat each day?
   At least 4 servings   =   0 points
   3 servings   =   1 point
   Less than 3 servings   =   4 points
        *Subscore*_____

(4) How many slices of whole-grain bread do you eat each
day?   At least 3 slices   =   0 points
   Less than 3 slices   =   4 points
        *Subscore*_____

(5) How many servings of rice, potatoes, or pasta do you
eat each day?
   At least 1 serving   =   0 points
   Less than 1 serving   =   4 points
        *Subscore*_____
        Your Score_____

f. Have you taken any positive steps to reduce your health risks?
 (1) How often do you use antioxidants?
   Regularly   =   0 points
   Sometimes   =   2 points
   Never   =   4 points
        *Subscore*_____

 (2) How often do you use meditation or some kind of mind
relaxation?
   Twice daily   =   0 points
   Once daily   =   1 point
   1 to 3 times/wk.   =   2 points
   Never   =   4 points
        *Subscore*_____

 (3) How often do you enjoy your hobbies (gardening, playing
the guitar, sailing, painting, etc.)?
   2+ times/wk.   =   0 points
   Once weekly   =   2 points
   Never   =   4 points
        *Subscore*_____
        Your Score_____

*YOUR TOTAL FOR SECTION 2*_____

Section 3 — Your General Cardiovascular Health

If it's been a while since you had a physical exam, you may need to visit a doctor or a medical laboratory for a simple blood test to get the answers to some of these questions.

a. What's your total cholesterol level?

160 or less	=	minus 2 points
161 to 179	=	0 points
180 to 209	=	1 point
210 to 219	=	2 points
220 to 239	=	4 points
240 to 259	=	6 points
260 or over	=	8 points
		Your Score_____

b. What's your high density lipoprotein (HDL) cholesterol level?

Male:	40 or over	=	0 points
	39 to 35	=	2 points
	34 to 30	=	4 points
	29 to 25	=	6 points
	Below 25	=	8 points
Female:	50 or over	=	0 points
	49 to 45	=	2 points
	44 to 40	=	4 points
	39 to 35	=	6 points
	Below 35	=	8 points
			Your Score_____

Divide your total cholesterol number by your HDL level to get your ratio of total cholesterol to HDL (ideally 4.5 or less)_____.

c. What's the level of your triglycerides (fasting for at least 8 hours prior to drawing blood)?

Below 100	=	0 points
100 to 151	=	1 point
151 to 300	=	2 points
Over 300	=	4 points
		Your Score_____

d. How's your blood pressure? (You can self-administer a blood pressure test using machines found in many drug stores.)

   (1) What's your systolic pressure?

Below 140	=	0 points
140 to 149	=	1 point
150 to 159	=	2 points
160 to 169	=	4 points
170 to 175	=	6 points
176 or over	=	8 points

*Subscore*_____

   (2) What's your diastolic pressure?

85 or below	=	0 points
86 to 90	=	1 point
91 to 95	=	2 points
96 to 100	=	4 points
101 to 105	=	6 points
Higher than 105	=	8 points

*Subscore*_____

Your Score_____

e. How's your heart?

   (1) Do you have heart disease?

No	=	0 points
Yes	=	4 points

*Subscore*_____

   (2) Do you have normal stress test results?

Yes	=	0 points
No	=	4 points
No test	=	0 points

*Subscore*_____

   (3) Do you have a normal EKG?:

Yes	=	0 points
No	=	2 points
No test	=	0 points

*Subscore*_____

Your Score_____

*YOUR TOTAL FOR SECTION 3*_____

Add your total scores from Sections 1, 2, and 3 to get
Your Grand Total:_____

Evaluate the Results of Your Assessment

While some health-risk assessments are read by computers and used to give a forecast of how long (statistically) the person being tested can expect to live, that's not our main purpose in administering this test. You can, however, rate yourself on your current chances of achieving healthy longevity by looking at your grand total score.

If your grand total is below 20, you're already doing many of the things that will guarantee you a long and healthy life. You're to be congratulated, but there's more you can do by focusing your attention on those parts of the assessment in which you amassed points.

If your score is in the 20 to 60 range, the range in which most people fall before they begin exercising and eating right and taking advantage of the benefits of antioxidants, your life span should be (all other things being equal) right around normal. Don't congratulate yourself, however. Remember, your goal is to move far, far beyond "normal" in terms of life expectancy. You'll do this by following my step-by-step program as outlined in this book.

If your score is 60 or higher, you are (as you probably know) acting in ways virtually guaranteed to shorten your life — and not taking actions that can guarantee longevity. However, don't panic! To be sure, you need to make changes in the way you live. But, even if your score is 90, my seven-step program will add decades to your life. In fact, as soon as you start actively practicing what you read in these pages, your score will begin to plummet.

Remember, the primary purpose of this self-test is to point out areas of your life in which you can effect change to live longer and healthier. With that in mind, let's examine each section of your assessment in turn.

Section 1: Your Family History

As I said earlier, if you have a family history of heart attack, cancer or diabetes, you're not "predestined" to die from or be debilitated by that disease. However, if you have a family history of heart attack, diabetes, or cancer (especially if your score is a "2" on sections 1a, 1b, or 1c of the assessment), it is critically important for you to control the major risk factors for your health.

1. Exercise regularly.
2. Avoid foods high in saturated fat and animal protein.
3. Eat a high-fiber diet (plenty of fruits and vegetables).

4. Undertake a program of stress management. Meditation, improved spirituality, happy relationships, hobbies, and time spent "playing" all reduce your risk factors here.

In addition:

5. Keep your body fat stable (16% is ideal for a man — 20% for a woman).
6. Have a stress test each year or two if you're over the age of 40 (male) or 50 (female).
7. Try to maintain a total cholesterol level of less than 180.
8. Take B vitamins like Niacin (500 to 1500 milligrams of slow release daily).
9. If natural ways to control your cholesterol fail, take prescription drugs as prescribed by your doctor.
10. Take antioxidant vitamins twice daily. Use co-enzyme Q-10 (a naturally occurring antioxidant) and herbs to neutralize free radical damage. (For specifics on vitamin and antioxidant doses, see Chapter Six.)
11. Finally, use the balance of this book as the basis for a long-term plan to make slow but steady changes in the way you live — changes that will guarantee you better health, more vitality and strength, and ultimate longevity.

Section 2: Your Lifestyle

Your ideal and ultimate goal should be a total score of "0" on this section of the assessment. But you won't, unless you're a paragon of healthy living, have that low score to begin with. You must work to achieve that healthy lifestyle.

If your behavior-risk score is a 50 (as high as possible for this section), it goes without saying that you need to make changes to mitigate the effects of your lifestyle choices on your health. Fortunately, even relatively minor changes will result in big drops in your score (and in big health benefits).

You can't change your heredity — you're stuck with your family medical history. You can, though, change your behavior to minimize your health risk and reverse some or all the damage you've already done. Consider the following:

1. *Smoking.* Smoking is linked to a variety of diseases including cancer, hypertension, and emphysema. The most common cause of death following surgery is lung problems,

usually linked to smoking. If you're an otherwise healthy 35-year-old who stops smoking, you'll add about seven years to your life!

If smoking is a problem for you — and I know it's one of the toughest of all addictions to break — consider asking your doctor for a prescription for one of the new smoke-cessation patches and a program to quit smoking. Hundreds of my patients have had great success using these patches to break their nicotine addictions when they combined the patches with hypnotherapy, meditation, and exercise. It has been my experience that not one thing, but a combination of efforts is necessary to break the smoking addiction. (See Special Supplement I on smoking cessation at the end of this book.)

2. *Alcohol abuse.* Alcohol abuse causes liver damage, hypertension, coronary artery disease (CAD), brain damage, damage to the pancreas and, of course, is a contributing factor in about half of all automobile accidents, injuries, and deaths every year. Though not scored in your Health-Risk Assessment, you need to determine if drinking is a problem for you. Even if you're not a "problem drinker" and you stop drinking, you'll gain at least a full year of life. If you're an alcohol abuser — that is, if alcohol is causing you problems at home, on your job, or with the law — when you quit, you gain as much as 15 years of life!

   (If you believe you are addicted to alcohol and can't stop drinking without help, I recommend contacting Alcoholics Anonymous.)

3. *Diet.* Eating foods high in fats and animal protein is a causative factor in diseases ranging from hypertension and coronary artery disease to cancer of the stomach, breast, prostate, and colon. In fact, diet is implicated as a leading culprit in as many as half of all heart attack and cancer deaths in the U.S. every year. A healthy diet will add about 10 years to your life!

4. *Exercise.* Many people don't make the time to exercise, even though studies have shown that a lack of exercise leads to increased risk of heart disease, stroke, hypertension, premature aging, osteoporosis (bone mineral loss), obesity,

arthritis, diabetes, and stress-related illnesses. (Stress itself can reduce your body's immunity and lead to other diseases.) Regular, moderate exercise, will add about five years
to your life!

Remember, while I urge and strongly advocate that you totally
eliminate the risks you uncover with your Health-Risk Assessment
(smoking or a fat-laden diet, for example), I understand that some
people either won't or can't give up the habits or addictions of a
lifetime. At least not easily. If you, for whatever reasons, decide
you just have to continue smoking, drinking, not exercising, etc.,
you can still mitigate or minimize the risks associated with your
decisions. My seven-step program for a century of great health
still offers you ways to extend your life and make your life healthier
by neutralizing some of the negative effects of your lifestyle.

Section 3: Your Cardiovascular Health

This section of the Health-Risk Assessment looks at factors
that could be an indication of heart attack or stroke.

As was the case with Section 2, your ultimate goal here should
be as low a cumulative score as possible (a "-2") when you assess
your overall cardiovascular health. Any higher score is a clear and
certain indication that you need to make changes in terms of diet,
exercise, and behavior to lower your cholesterol levels, raise your
HDL count so that your ratio of total cholesterol is 4.5 or less,
lower your triglyceride level, and lower your blood pressure rate to
within a healthy range.

If you have heart disease, don't despair. We know we can reverse as well as prevent heart disease. Exercise, cardiac rehabilitation, meditation, yoga, a low-fat vegetarian diet, and stress management are all major ways to reduce your cardiovascular risks.

Cholesterol

Your total cholesterol is made up of both high density lipoprotein (HDL) and low density lipoprotein (LDL). The HDL protects
you from heart disease. That's why, ideally, it should be higher
than 40 in a man and higher than 50 in a woman. On the other
hand, your LDL should be as low as possible. The LDL is heavier
and adds deposits to the lining of the wall of the arteries, leading to
atherosclerosis (hardening of the arteries).

Think of it like this: LDL is like dust that clings to your carpet. HDL is like a vacuum that sucks the dust off your carpet.

To keep your HDL level high, avoid smoking, exercise regularly (at least three times a week), keep your body fat at 16% (for men) and 20% (for women), and control the effects of stress in your life.

LDL is controlled with diet. If your LDL and total cholesterol are high, then a diet of 10% fat, 75% carbohydrate (complex), and 15% protein (from vegetables only) will lower your total cholesterol and LDL at the same time.

Triglycerides

Triglycerides fluctuate much more than cholesterol. The predominant source of triglycerides is simple sugars. The worst offender is a simple sugar known as alcohol. Even though people with high triglycerides are told to avoid fruit, they should ignore that recommendation. It is true that fruit can raise your triglyceride levels. However, the benefits of the phytochemicals, minerals, and antioxidants in fruit offset the moderate rise in triglyceride levels.

My Seven-Step Program
for a Century of Great Health

My seven-step program is designed — as you'll see while you progress through the program — to address any and all of the danger signals sent aloft by your Health-Risk Assessment. To mitigate the risk associated with a family history of life-threatening or debilitating illness. To give you both the impetus and the means to change your unhealthy behaviors. To turn back the hands of time and actually reverse damage done to your body by the lifestyle choices you've made over the years.

In coming chapters, I'll give you all the tools you need to change your life, and to develop your own plan for healthy longevity. You'll find out just what to do, and how, so that your next Health-Risk Assessment will paint a portrait of a healthy individual well on the way to a longer, healthier, and happier life.

Proceed through the balance of my seven-step program at your own pace. However, keep in mind that this is a long-range program, and it may take you several years before you have made all seven steps habits in your life.

Recognize that it takes at least nine months (and as long a 18 months) for any individual to become habituated to a new way of living. If you are a smoker, for example, it will take from nine months to 18 months for you to become an habitual non-smoker.

Also, understand that you shouldn't try to change more than one major area of your life at a time. People who try to change too much at one time almost invariably fail. The best path to success is to wait until you have moved at least part way along one path — from habitual smoking to habitual non-smoking, for example — before you make another major change.

Does this mean that if you're trying to stop smoking you shouldn't do anything else to improve your life for at least nine months? No, not at all. In fact, as you'll see in the next chapter, there are some steps in my seven-step program that you will most likely take simultaneously. That does not negate the fact, however, that you should not try to change everything all at once.

Only you will know when you are ready to take the next step. I can't give you solid rules on how quickly to proceed. Take exercise, for example. Once you start a program of aerobics, it may take you a full year or more to become an habitual exerciser. You may be comfortable doing aerobics plus practicing some formal method of stress management after just a few weeks or months. However, you may want to wait a year before moving on. It is up to you. You have the freedom to move at your own pace. You have no reason to feel guilty if it takes you three or four or even five years to become completely habituated to your new way of life.

I know you want to achieve perfect health today. That you want to put the entire program for healthy longevity to work right now. But I urge you to be patient. My experience with my own life and with patients in my Florida clinic has shown me over and over again that slow and steady progress, over time, is a better and more certain path to ultimate success.

Later in this book, I'll talk specifically about exercises — both aerobics and weight training — you can use to strengthen your heart, lungs, bones, and muscles, about stress-reduction techniques (including meditation), and about ways you can change your diet to lose weight and feel great without feeling hungry all the time. For now, though, remember to be gentle and patient with yourself as you begin to modify your life.

Chapter Six

Step 2:
The Most Important Medical
Discovery of Our Time

The most important medical discovery of the last half-century concerns two substances called "free radicals" and "antioxidants." Free radicals have been linked to (at last count) about 60 diseases. And we now have evidence that antioxidants can protect against, stop, and (in some instances) even reverse the damage done by free radicals.

These discoveries are as important to the health and well-being of men and women all around the world as was the discovery of penicillin or the discovery that simple sterilization techniques would stop infection in operating rooms.

These discoveries make clear that the most important single thing you can do if you want to live long enough to dance the polka at your great-great-grandson's wedding is start an immediate regimen to make sure you get all the antioxidants you need — both through diet and through the use of nutrients and dietary supplements.

63

A theory that's been around for 40 years

If, like most people, you've gotten whatever information you have about free radicals and antioxidants from the popular press and television, you probably think free radicals were just discovered a few months or even weeks ago. In fact, the theory that free radicals are linked to aging and death was first put forward about 40 years ago by Dr. Denham Harman of the University of Nebraska.

At that time, Dr. Harman's theory was viewed by some to be the product of a crack-pot mind. At best, it was considered to be little more than another interesting hypothesis in a field (gerontology, or the study of aging) that has long been filled with hypotheses.

An interesting hypothesis was largely what it remained until the last decade or so when an increasing number of scientists started their own experiments into the causes and prevention of aging. Those experiments, in turn, have produced growing enthusiasm for the propositions first put forward by Dr. Harman almost 40 years ago.

Until very recently, much of the experimental laboratory work undertaken to find out exactly how and why free radicals scavenge the body, and — more important — how we can ward off their attacks, has been largely unreported in the non-scientific press. Findings went unreported, even though research was indicating clear evidence — first, of a link between free radicals and aging, and second, of the ability of antioxidants to stop or reverse free radical damage.

Why isn't this news being shouted from the rooftops?

If these studies have been ongoing, why are most people only now beginning to learn about free radicals and antioxidants?

The medical community is ultra-conservative when it comes to making new ideas and new therapies available to the public. There are, I believe, several reasons for this conservatism. Some of them are laudable, and some are regrettable. On the one hand, for example, scientists want to be 100-percent certain of their findings before they release them. Wrong conclusions can have tragic consequences. On the other hand, scientists can have a "blind spot" when it comes to any discoveries that challenge long-accepted beliefs.

This ultra-conservatism, while often justified — particularly in the case of a new drug therapy or invasive surgical procedure that could be harmful to patients — can be carried to extremes. And that, in my estimation, is exactly what's happening with research into free radicals and antioxidants. The medical community — not entirely, but in the main — is being overly conservative by not trumpeting the news that you can, indeed, expect to live to be 120 if you take some relatively simple steps. It's dragging its feet even in the face of what I view as overwhelming evidence linking free radicals to aging and death — and linking antioxidants to longer, healthier life spans.

Common sense vs. "gold standard" of evidence

Unfortunately, most of the evidence uncovered so far has not been the result of traditional research methods. Instead, it is what we might call "commonsense evidence." A study of a large group of nurses at the Harvard School of Public Health, for example, showed that taking 100 I.U.s (international units) of vitamin E daily reduced the risk of heart disease in those nurses by almost 50 percent. Common sense, then, would indicate that taking the antioxidant vitamin E would, at the very least, help lower your risk of heart attack. This evidence though, was not the product of what one researcher called the "gold standard" of medical research. It was not the result of a controlled clinical trial — a study conducted on a large population with two groups of individuals randomly selected either to receive vitamin E, or to receive no supplement, or to receive a placebo over a long period of time. So, since the "gold standard" of research was not used, the results of the Harvard School study — and others — are largely overlooked or discounted by most in the medical community.

This means that the medical community, as a whole, won't come out and openly endorse the idea that free radicals are the agents of aging, disease, and death until the evidence of randomized clinical studies is so staggering that it can no longer be questioned on any level. And that's likely to take at least another decade.

In the meantime, of course, people are growing older and weaker. They're suffering from disease and illness — and they're dying from a lack of available information. With that in mind, I urge you to pay close attention to the information that follows.

You need the very latest information

I'll admit, up front and at the outset, that the information I'm going to give you about free radicals isn't exact or complete. Research scientists around the world and practitioners like me are uncovering and discovering new facts each and every day. What I'm putting in your hands is the very latest information that's available today. It will be up to you to stay abreast of breaking news from the front in the war against aging and death. You'll be able to do this by reading a handful of publications that bring you the latest scientific medical findings in a way that you can use them. These include my newsletter, "Health & Longevity," *Longevity* magazine, and *Prevention* magazine.

Your only other choice is to wait the 10 years or more it will take for the medical community to jump on the free radical/antioxidant bandwagon. You can wait for a final okay from the American Medical Association before you take action to stop the damage being done to your body every day by free radicals. However, it is my belief that if you delay and don't take the few simple actions I'll tell you about to stop free radicals cold — and even reverse the damage they've already done to your body — you'll be turning your back on the greatest preventive-therapeutic tool in the history of medicine.

Just what are free radicals?

You need to know a bit more about free radicals and how they attack the body before you can wage your own personal war against these agents of age and illness. So, before we talk about how antioxidants can serve as both preventive and therapeutic tools, let's take a look at exactly what free radicals are and how they lead to aging, disease, and death. And let's take a look at some specific free radical/antioxidant studies.

To get a better idea of what free radicals are and how they cause destruction, try to imagine a Viking horde at work inside your body. Imagine this army attacking and damaging healthy cells, breaking down the collagen that keeps your skin firm and youthful, attacking your eyes so that you develop cataracts, working away inside your circulatory system to cause heart disease and stroke, joining forces with cigarette smoke to increase your risk of lung cancer (if you're a smoker), and so on.

That's a simple way to visualize free radicals.

In more scientific terms, free radicals are highly unstable oxygen molecules created as a by-product of normal metabolism. Unlike a stable molecule that has electrons that are paired so that their positive and negative electrical charges are canceled out (neutral), a free radical has an unpaired electrically charged fragment that is hungry for a mate. So, free radicals do their damage by "stealing" electrons from stable molecules. This turns these molecules into new free radicals that prey on other stable molecules — and so on. As a result, normal body structures break down and don't reconstruct. Free radicals can puncture cell membranes, allowing fluids to leak out and disrupting the ability of the cell to take in nutrients. They can even break up the body's DNA and RNA — the basic building blocks of genetics — creating mutations that reproduce uncontrollably.

A destructive chain reaction

Dr. Harman, who first proposed the free radical theory of aging, likened the way free radicals work in the body to a chain reaction of linked, destructive activity. You can see a free radical destructive chain reaction at work by cutting an apple in half. After a few minutes, you'll see the apple start to turn brown. What you're watching here is the process of free radicals attacking and changing the molecular structure of the fruit by "stealing" electrons from healthy molecules.

However, if you put the juice of a lemon (which is loaded with vitamin C) on the cut surfaces of the apple, you will neutralize the process — or at least slow it down — and get a first-hand look at how antioxidants (like vitamin C) work.

Brown, discolored fruit is, at worst, distasteful. But what free radicals do in your body is downright deadly.

A deadly dilemma

This presents us with what can truly be viewed as a deadly dilemma. Oxygen, after all, is necessary for life. It is fuel for your cells, and your body can't function without it. At the same time, that life-sustaining oxygen in your system is creating cell-destroying free radicals.

However, every organism that depends on oxygen for fuel has a built-in system to diffuse the damage done by that oxygen. Ducks and mice and other animals with relatively short life spans have relatively ineffective systems for dealing with free radical damage. Humans, though, with the potential of living well over 100 years, are better equipped.

Our bodies fight free radicals three ways

It appears that we have, in fact, three lines of defense against free radical damage.

1. Our first line of defense is our own enzyme system. We have three enzymes in our bodies that function as antioxidants by tearing free radicals apart and rendering them harmless — superoxide dismutase (SOD), catalase, and glutathione peroxidase. SOD and glutathione peroxidase provide the most effective protection. If medical scientists could manufacture these enzymes in the laboratory and produce them in pill form, aging could be slowed to a crawl, and many of the diseases that now routinely shorten life would be conquered.

2. Our second line of defense is provided by an internal system that creates biologic molecules that give up electrons to the hungry free radicals. Less crucial cells are sacrificed, but crucial cells are protected. This system does not work as well as the enzyme system. It neutralizes the free radicals, but it changes the optimum function of the body's cells in the process.

3. Our final line of defense is found in nutrients that neutralize free radicals, but sacrifice themselves. For example, vitamin E (one of these nutrients) can attach itself to a free radical and neutralize the free radical so it can't do any damage. However, sometimes in this process, the vitamin E itself becomes a free radical. A Reactive Oxygen Species (ROS) is created which has a free electron and can cause damage.

This last line of defense is obviously not as efficient as the first — the body's own natural enzyme system. But, for now, the use of nutrients (both those found in foods and in supplements) is the best way I know of to intervene and disrupt the process of destruction that is caused by free radicals.

The next wave of research

My belief is that the next wave of research on disease prevention should focus either on stimulating the body's natural production of SOD, catalase, and glutathione peroxidase, or on synthesizing these enzymes so they can be taken in pill form. True healing will ultimately stem from this kind of research.

If we are successful in controlling free radicals, we could change the course of medical history. Free radicals are all around and inside all of us. Thousands and thousands of these tiny marauders wander through our cells, leaving pockets of damage in their wake. Scientists know from recent research that even breathing and drinking water promote free radical formation, and that the food we eat cannot be metabolized (used by the body) without free radical activity.

The body does have natural defenses against free radicals, but those defenses are not limitless. When the body produces more free radicals than these defenses can handle (because of poor diet, smoking, exposure to environmental pollutants, and other causes), those defenses are simply overwhelmed.

The link between free radicals and specific diseases

Let's look at just a few diseases — diseases that not only kill, but also make life painful — and see what scientific research says about the involvement of free radicals.

• *Heart Disease.* Researchers now have proven that free radicals attack so-called "bad" cholesterol (LDL, or low-density lipoprotein), and oxidize it into a form that damages the lining of the coronary arteries. The body, in response, patches the damaged arterial lining by forming plaque (a fatty deposit) that narrows the arteries, and ultimately leads to heart disease.

• *Stroke.* Just as a build-up of plaque in the coronary arteries leads to heart attack, so a build-up of this gunk in cerebral arteries can lead to what doctors euphemistically call a "cerebral accident" — a stroke. Scientists haven't yet officially connected this type of build-up to free radicals, but it makes sense to me — common sense — that if free radicals cause plaque in coronary arteries, they'll cause the same kind of plaque formation in other arteries.

All strokes are not due to a build-up of plaque in the arteries in or to the brain. There's no doubt that free radicals do damage to the vessel walls — and a damaged arterial wall can bleed into the brain, causing a stroke.

• *Cancer.* Scientists know that free radicals have the ability to change a cell's DNA in a way that can make healthy cells become cancerous. They also know that although the body has natural defenses against the free radicals that constantly bombard our cells, the unstopped free radical damage that occurs when these natural defenses have been overwhelmed has been linked to breast, lung, and colon cancers — three cancers that account for about half of all cancer deaths in the U.S. each year.

• *Cataracts and other age-related conditions.* While there has not yet been any firm proof, scientists believe that free radical damage is responsible for many other diseases and conditions long thought to be a "normal" part of the aging process. Included in the long and growing list of problems with a suspected free radical link are cataracts (free radical damage associated with light rays), wrinkling and skin discoloration (free radical damage associated with exposure to the sun) — even senility (free radical damage associated with diet). Diabetes, inflammatory bowel disease, pancreatitis (inflammation of the pancreas), and peptic ulcers also may be linked to free radical damage.

Don't wait

Scientists will give us the official word on the cause-and-effect relationship between free radicals and disease in 10 years or so. But I'm not willing to wait that long. And you shouldn't be willing to wait either, because there are things you can do — today — to combat any possible damage being done by free radicals in your body. You can take action today that will — I believe with all my heart — not only give you protection from a wide variety of illnesses and debilitating conditions associated with aging, but also will ward off and even reverse the damage done by these voracious agents of age and decay.

Antioxidants to the rescue!

Research has shown that antioxidants rush to do battle with the marauding army of free radicals that attack our healthy cells. And we know that antioxidants — readily available from natural food sources and from dietary supplements and vitamins — have the ability to defeat free radicals in the body.

Theories abound concerning just how and why antioxidants fight aging and disease. Some of the most intriguing ongoing research — being conducted by the National Institute on Aging — indicates that when a cell line (the multi-generational "family" of cells that's

formed as cells divide and re-divide over time) is young, the enzymes we know as antioxidants naturally disarm and make harmless free radicals. Over time, though, these enzymes appear to lose
their ability to counteract the effects of free radicals. This leads to
aging and, ultimately, death. In other words, as your body's cells
age, your natural antioxidants need reinforcements in their battle
against rampaging free radicals.

This same research already has shown that longer-lived species have more naturally occurring antioxidants in their bodies than
do shorter-lived animals. This gives even more credence to the importance of antioxidants in the fight for a longer, healthier life.

Up-to-the-minute research

As I write this chapter, more scientific evidence is being presented showing the link between free radicals and aging and disease — and also showing how antioxidants can break that link and
actually stop the aging process. One study, undertaken by Dr.
Rajindar Sohal and Dr. William Orr, biologists at Southern Meth-
odist University, published results in the journal *Science* in late
February 1994. This study provided what Sohal said was the "first
direct" evidence that free radicals cause aging, and that the use of
antioxidants can stop that process.

In the Sohal-Orr study, fruit flies were given extra copies of
genes (the enzyme SOD to convert free radicals to hydrogen peroxide, and the enzyme catalase to convert hydrogen peroxide to
water) that normally work in the body to rid cells of free radicals.
The result was truly remarkable. The flies that were given the extra genes lived 30 percent longer than those that did not receive the
genes. In addition, according to the researchers, the genetically
altered fruit flies were more spry, vigorous, and nimble while they
were alive. In other words, they stayed younger.

In fact, said Sohal, "We could tell which ones [were given the
free radical fighting genes] just by looking at them."

To be sure, this experiment was on fruit flies, not humans.
However, humans and flies have almost identical systems for dealing with and defusing free radicals.

Three ways to boost your antioxidant levels

I can't alter my genes, or yours, to extend life (though that may be an option in the future). I can, though, tell you how to boost your antioxidant levels, starting today, in order to add healthy years to your life by combating the effects of free radicals.

1. Take antioxidant vitamins and mineral supplements with the proven ability to protect your body against the ravages of free radicals. These include vitamins E, C, A, beta-carotene, and the mineral nutrients selenium, glutathione, and pycnogenal.

Though there is still controversy about how effective antioxidant vitamins are, and just how much protection they ultimately provide, I believe they're among your best defenses against age and disease. I am not saying that vitamins alone are the answer. If you smoke, for example, do not expect a vitamin to protect you against lung cancer. However, if you quit smoking, plus improve your diet, plus take antioxidant vitamins, you can repair damage done by smoking and protect yourself against cancer. If you take antioxidants in conjunction with the dietary recommendations I'll give you later in this book, you will have a real and substantially lower risk of premature aging and disease.

2. Change your diet to provide yourself not only with the vitamins and minerals you need for health, but to furnish your body with the naturally occurring antioxidant phytochemicals found in certain foods. Phytochemicals are complex substances like sulforaphane (present in broccoli) that sweep carcinogens (cancer causing agents) out of the cells.

Think of them as elements that naturally occur in organic foods to protect against cancer-causing agents that damage cells. Think of them as a natural way to keep cancer cells from multiplying — an organic way to keep cancer from shortening your life.

Intense study of phytochemicals has just begun, but already we have found benefits from phytochemicals like flavonoids in citrus fruits and berries, P-courmaric acid and cholorogenic acid in tomatoes, allylic sulfides in garlic and onions, capsaicin in chili peppers, and genisterin in soybeans.

Vegetables, fruits, grains, onions, and garlic ward off cancer by providing as many of the naturally occurring antioxidant phytochemicals as you can possibly get from food sources. These foods are also high in fiber, and thus afford protection against colon cancer, breast cancer, and all types of intestinal cancer.

I advocate a diet high in freshly grown fruits, vegetables, and grains. This diet, similar to the diet eaten by our ancestors, will help give you additional antioxidant chemical protection. (I'll tell you more about diet and nutrition later.)

3. Start using antioxidant herbs, in moderation. They can be used as food flavorings, in herbal teas, or in capsule, tincture, or freeze-dried doses. The following herbs are known to be high in antioxidant properties: rosemary, lemon balm, thyme, oregano, sage, ginger, garlic, turmeric, and echinacea. Other spices believed by some experts to promote antioxidant activity include basil, allspice, lemon grass, mace, nutmeg, celery seed, black pepper, hot chili peppers, cloves, capsicum, cumin, and alfalfa leaves.

Herbal remedies have been used for centuries in other cultures, but have been generally ignored by the Western medical establishment. Recently, however, even the most conservative researchers have started to take note of the time-proven benefits of medicinal plants. Scientists are journeying into rain forests, to the Himalayas, to the Indian tribes of Peru to study ancient herbal treatments still used by "medicine men" and "shamans." Because they work.

In a recently published textbook, *Freedom From Disease*, Hari Sharma, M.D., a professor of Pathology at the Ohio State University College of Medicine, reported on a multi-university project he had organized to study Indian herbs. Dr. Sharma's research identified three ancient, herbal preparations — an herbal nectar (called Maharishi Amrit Kalash, or MAK), an herbal mixture (called MA 631), and an herbal tea (called Raja's Cup) — that are at least 1,000 times more potent than vitamins C and E as free radical scavengers. Dr. Sharma also discovered that two ancient herbal remedies — Amrit Nectar (MAK-4) and Ambrosia (MAK-5) — greatly increase the responsiveness of the immune system. They reduced the free radical damage produced when a potent anti-cancer drug (adriamycin) was given to both animals and humans.

We are, today, on the leading edge of a new practice of medicine — 21st century medicine. At last, the wisdom of the ages will be combined with the modern technology developed by some of the world's greatest scientific minds to unlock the keys to healthy life well beyond the age of 100.

The value of antioxidants to prevent disease

The efficacy of antioxidants — both from supplements and from herbal preparations — to prevent disease is beyond question. Let's examine a few specific examples.

    1. *Heart Attack.*

    • A joint study by the Harvard School of Public Health and Boston's Brigham and Women's Hospital tracked the course of more than 87,000 women and 45,000 men who had no history of heart disease to see if taking the antioxidant vitamin E would have any effect on their risk of developing the disease. The bottom line? Women who took more than 100 I.U.s of vitamin E for more than two years had about half the risk of heart disease as women who didn't. Men who took the same dose over the same period reduced their risk by more than 25 percent.

    • Researchers at Loma Linda University studied the connection between diet and death in 27,529 California Seventh Day Adventist adults over a period of two decades. The Adventists made nearly perfect research subjects since they follow strict dietary practices that set them apart from the general U.S. population. They are prohibited from eating pork and drinking alcoholic beverages, for example, and are urged not to eat meat, fish, or eggs, not to smoke or drink coffee, and to avoid spices.

    That survey showed, beyond any doubt, that a vegetarian diet — which is loaded with antioxidants that protect against free radicals — resulted in lower death rates in both men and women for coronary disease.

    Don't let the idea of a vegetarian diet scare you into closing this book. While I advocate that you limit the amount of animal protein you take in each and every day, I am not a strict adherent of vegetarianism. It is important to remember, though, that there is a relationship between a diet high in fat and the risk of death due to heart disease. That when you cook, fat becomes even more deadly because fat molecules, when heated, start to oxidize even before they get into your body. And that a diet filled with vegetables and low in animal fat will help you avoid what Harry Demopoulos, M.D., co-author of *Formula for Life — the Anti-Oxidant, Free Radical Detoxification Program*, calls "the free radical mess."

    2. *Stroke.*

    • The Harvard Medical School/Boston Hospital study mentioned above also showed that women who ate five or more servings per week of carrots (one of the vegetables high in the antioxidants vitamin C and beta-carotene) had a 68 percent lower risk of stroke than women who ate no more than one serving per month.

• Another study, conducted at the University of Tennessee in Memphis, showed that men and women who had the highest intake of vitamin E had the least thickening of the walls of the arteries leading to the brain, and, thus, a significantly lower risk of stroke.

3. *Senility.*

• A National Academy of Science study showed that administering the antioxidant agent PBN to old gerbils decreased the amount of free radical damaged tissue in the animals' brains and actually reversed memory loss (as measured by a maze test). In fact, after two weeks of treatment with PBN, the old gerbils in the test had mental acuity similar to that of young animals. In addition, once the PBN was discontinued, the animals rapidly started aging once again.

This is an example of the kind of study that many in the medical community would say has little, if any, relevance to us. After all, gerbils aren't humans. But I believe that the results of this study lead straight to the commonsense conclusion that if I boost my antioxidant intake, through diet and dietary supplements, I will be able to ward off the effects of aging.

4. *Cancer.*

• A study conducted by the National Cancer Institute (NCI) found that people who regularly took 100 I.U.s of vitamin E supplements, along with other supplements, had about half the risk of developing cancer of the mouth and throat than those who did not take the vitamin E supplements.

• Another study — of 30,000 Chinese men and women — that was jointly sponsored by the NCI and several Chinese medical research institutions, showed that individuals who were given daily doses of vitamin E and the mineral selenium along with beta-carotene over a five-year period showed a decrease of 13 percent in their overall cancer risk compared with the risk of a group given placebos. Of even more interest to researchers, those in the group who received beta-carotene had a 21 percent reduction in stomach cancer risk. (Stomach cancer is the most common form of cancer in China). These results, researchers noted, might have been slightly skewed because the general nutritional levels of those in the study

were improved as part of the study. However, the results offer real
hope that vitamins and minerals may be effective in reducing cancer.

   • Still another study showed that daily doses of beta-carotene
actually had the ability to heal mouth lesions (growths) in some
cigarette smokers — and that those lesions would reappear once
the beta-carotene intake stopped.

   • The Loma Linda study cited above also pointed out the
value of a vegetarian diet (a diet rich in antioxidants and
phytochemicals) in battling cancer. Both male and female vegetarians in that study had lower death rates for colon cancer, and
the women had lower death rates for ovarian cancer.

   It is these studies — and many other studies like them —
showing the ability of vitamins, nutrients, and herbs to counteract
the damaging effects of free radicals that lead me to trumpet the
discovery of antioxidants as the "most important health discovery
of the past 50 years!"

Put antioxidants to work for you

   If you want to put antioxidants to work in your body — and I
must say again that this is the single most important step you can
take to promote your own health and to guarantee yourself good
health to the age of 100 — I urge you to start taking antioxidant
supplements now.

   In fact, if you take no other action as a result of reading this
book, at least boost your antioxidant levels. You will see almost
immediate, visible, tangible evidence that these substances are
working to protect you from free radical damage. Patients who
take this advice report increased energy, positive changes in skin
texture, and even loss of wrinkles — within a few weeks.

   And — please — if you simply must smoke and eat fatty foods
and continue other behaviors that promote free radical damage, at
least be aware of the risks you run. Mitigate those risks as much as
possible by taking antioxidant vitamins and supplements, and by
eating a diet rich in antioxidant vegetables (red, orange, and yellow) and herbs.

   It is also important for you to realize that as soon as this book
goes into print, new information will become available and that is
why my newsletter, "Health & Longevity," exists: to give you the
very latest information.

There are many, many antioxidants — not just those that I have been telling you about. For example, I have not discussed the co-enzyme Q-10, the amino acids L carnitine and L lysine, and many other agents that are often present naturally in high fiber, low fat diets that are based on organic vegetables and grains. However, my purpose here is to get you started on a regular course of action. Over time, you may want to experiment with additional supplements and "fine tune" your own dietary program according to your own individual needs.

Actions to Take

• Vitamin A. Take up to, but no more than, 10,000 I.U.s daily. (Vitamin A can be toxic in larger doses.)

• Beta-Carotene (the water soluble precursor of vitamin A). Take 12,000 to 25,000 I.U.s daily.

• Vitamin E. Take 400 to 800 I.U.s per day. (This is a conservative recommended dose that may be pushed higher as research indicates.)

• Vitamin C. Take 500 to 2,000 milligrams daily. There's no "ideal" dose for vitamin C at the current time. You'll know you're taking too much if you begin to suffer from diarrhea or flatulence. If that happens, cut back on your dosage.

You can bolster the effect of vitamin C by taking pycnogenal, a special blend of a type of bioflavonoid called proanthocyanidins. This strong antioxidant prevents vitamin C from being oxidized and helps it act as an enzyme-ascorbic oxidase.

• Trace Minerals, Amino Acids, and Enzymes. Take 200 micrograms of selenium, 40 to 100 milligrams of glutathione, 40 to 100 milligrams of pycnogenal, and 60 to 120 milligrams of co-enzyme Q-10 a day. These substances are not included in multivitamins. Purchase them separately.

The trace mineral selenium is particularly important since it plays a major role in disease prevention as a component in the glutathione system. It appears, in fact, that people who live in areas where the soil has been depleted of selenium may actually be more susceptible to disease. In South Dakota, for example, where the selenium level of the soil is among the highest in the nation, cancer levels are among the lowest. And in Ohio, where soil is largely selenium-depleted, there is a much higher incidence of cancer. Individuals with high levels of selenium in their blood have low cancer rates — and a low level of selenium in the blood indicates cancer risk.

• Herbal Preparations. While there are literally thousands of herbal preparations available from both Western and Eastern herbologists, I have found Dr. Sharma's research to be very convincing. (See page 73.) In light of his research, I recommend that you take daily doses of MAK-4 and MAK-5.

Chapter Seven

Step 3:
The Breath of Life

I very strongly believe that exercise is a preventive and healing medicine for both the mind and the body. Eastern cultures have known this for centuries. In our culture — and in my seven-step program — we use different kinds of exercises to achieve different results: aerobics for endurance, weight training for strength, and stretching exercises for flexibility. However, in India, China, and Japan, our counterparts are able to increase flexibility, endurance, and strength — all at the same time — through the mind-body control of the ancient arts of yoga, t'ai chi, karate, and judo.

We are still evolving toward achieving such balance and unity, though we are making more progress all the time. One of the leading researchers working to help us realize this goal is Dr. John Douillard.

A window to the future
In his hallmark book, *Body, Mind and Sport*, Dr. Douillard

shows how he has utilized his knowledge of Ayurvedic medicine, yoga, and aerobics to develop a technique to improve the way we exercise. He demonstrates that an individual who uses traditional mouth breathing when running or walking could have a heart rate of 170 to 180 and a breath rate of 30 to 50. But if that individual incorporates the yogic breathing style, he or she can perform the same run or walk at the same pace with a heart rate of 130 to 150 and a breathing rate of 12 to 18.

According to Dr. Douillard's system, the duration and frequency of the exercise depends on the runner's Ayurvedic mind-body type. For example, a thin, hyperactive, "vata" type would do less exercise than a stocky "kapha" type.

Striving for maximum benefits

The value of aerobics has been proven beyond any doubt. That's what makes it such an important component of my program. Study after study has shown that as soon as you start to exercise aerobically, your overall health will improve, you'll immediately begin to look better and younger, and you'll feel more vibrant and alive.

We have already learned many important things about aerobic exercise — that moderation is very important, that consistency yields much better results than intensity, and that more is not always better. Now we can learn from Dr. Douillard and work toward joining East and West to achieve the maximum benefits.

Even moderate exercise makes a difference

Recent studies show that an inactive lifestyle — too many hours spent as a "couch potato" and too few hours engaged in even simple exercise — contributes to about 250,000 deaths annually. And that people who don't exercise are twice as likely to suffer from heart disease as men and women who do exercise.

At the University of Utah Medical School, researchers found that regular participation in activities like walking, bowling, raking leaves, and ballroom dancing was enough to reduce the risk of heart attack by 30 percent. And the University of Wisconsin Medical School proved that heart attack patients who took part in a specially designed exercise program were able to reduce their death rate from coronary artery disease by 25 percent — about the same rate as could be achieved by drugs, but without any side-effects.

Other studies have shown that even moderate aerobic exercise — which I define as any activity that uses the large muscle groups of the body in a rhythmic fashion to deliver oxygen throughout the body as efficiently as possible — will help you avoid strokes, high blood pressure, muscle weakness and memory loss, osteoporosis, arthritis, and diabetes.

And that's not all. Exercise also reduces anxiety and tension, and gives a boost to the body's immune system.

Your heart needs to "breathe" too

Why is it that aerobic exercise is such a vitally important part of my seven-step program to a century of great health? What is it that aerobic exercise provides that no other form of exercise provides in the same way and to the same extent? Why do I believe that aerobic exercise is the most beneficial thing you can do for yourself?

The answer to these three questions can be summed up in one word: Oxygen. Oxygen is your body's fuel. Essentially, oxygen is to your body what gasoline is to an automobile. Stated as simply as possible, your lungs draw oxygen in, and your heart delivers that oxygen supply to every cell in your body, where it is used to create energy. The more efficient your heart is at delivering this fuel, the more oxygen your body will be able to consume, and the more energy you will have.

Measuring the heart's efficiency

Just as a car is fueled by gas, our bodies are fueled by oxygen. And the more efficient we are at using that fuel, the more work our bodies can do with less effort.

A simple measure of the heart's efficiency is found in the rate of the body's oxygen consumption in terms of milliliters (ml) per kilogram (kg) of body weight per minute (min). The average oxygen consumption for healthy women and men is about 35 to 40 ml/kg/min, while the oxygen consumption of a world-class endurance athlete (a triathlon competitor or a cross-country skier) may be as high as 65 to 80 ml/kg/min. Since there is a direct relationship between heart rate and oxygen delivery as the heart pumps more blood through the body, more oxygen is delivered.

An athlete using 40 ml/kg/min is working at only 47 to 60 percent of his or her maximum capability. Therefore, the heart rate of that athlete is much lower — and more efficient — than the heart rate of the average person exerting the same effort. The athlete is able to run both faster and farther, using the same amount of oxygen as the average person, but expending 40 to 50 percent less energy.

Everyone can benefit from aerobics

When we are young, most of us have bodies that are top-notch energy producers. We are able to obtain all the oxygen we need with a minimum of strain, and are able to turn that oxygen into energy so we can race and play tennis and mow the lawn, and hardly notice the effort. I say "most of us" because there are some who, for genetic reasons, have always been low energy producers — who have always had low oxygen consumption levels. For those few, exercise has always been a struggle.

Now, however, we know that everyone can improve his or her fuel efficiency — can boost his or her body's oxygen consumption level — simply by following a regimen of systematic aerobic exercise. That includes you, no matter what your current physical condition, and even if you are genetically predisposed to low oxygen consumption.

Reverse the symptoms of "old age"

If you feel the strain on your heart and lungs whenever you exert yourself, don't think that this is a symptom of "age" that you simply have to live with. That's not your problem. The problem is that you have allowed your body to become less efficient at obtaining the oxygen you need to produce energy.

Fortunately, this is a process that can be easily reversed with aerobic exercise. It can be reversed even if you've already started down the path to poor fitness. Even if you've moved far down the path.

Remember the work done by Fred Kasch at San Diego State University in which Kasch documented how a 61-year-old grandfather had the aerobic power (the ability of the body to get oxygen and oxygen-rich blood to all its organs) of a 25-year-old? And the 75-year-old who had better heart-lung capacity after taking part in Kasch's program than he did when he was 45?

Results like these are commonplace. And they can be yours — will be yours — provided you're willing to undertake a simple program of aerobic exercise. Aerobics will improve the efficiency of your heart and the ability of your lungs to extract oxygen from the environment. It will force your body to demand oxygen, process it, and deliver it to all your organs.

Set your sights high

You don't have to set your sights on competing in the next Olympics — but you can realistically boost your oxygen consumption close to that of a world-class athlete.

Here's a true story that will illustrate just what I mean:

Ken was a busy executive. Overweight and out-of-shape, he was too busy to take care of himself. At the age of 32, he had chest pains — and, ultimately, four heart bypasses. I met him when he was 36 years old and looking for a way to reduce the risk of having to undergo open heart surgery yet again.

Ken had never liked exercise. He had not been an athlete as a child or as a young man, always preferring to work with computers. But, as soon as Ken started the aerobics program I set up for him, he noticed dramatic results. Within just three months, his weight dropped form 232 pounds to 218, and he had more energy than he'd ever dreamed possible. Two years later, I set out to convince him to run in a 5-kilometer (3.1 mile) race.

At first, he was skeptical. "I could never do that," he said. "I've never run more than a few blocks in my life."

Finally, after a great deal of cajoling on my part, he agreed — and, after a few more months of aerobic training, I ran by his side in his first 5-kilometer race. By that time, he'd been running four days a week for three months and was down to 192 pounds. He was thrilled by the cheers of the crowd along the race course, by the attention of the media, and most of all by the proud looks he got from his family when he crossed the finish line. He had proved what the average person is capable of doing — even after open heart surgery.

The results of aerobics are immediate and dramatic

You can do what Ken did. You can start an aerobics program and almost immediately add years to your life with:

• A stronger, more efficient heart. When you're at rest, your heart rate will be about 10 to 20 beats-per-minute lower than the heart rate of an unconditioned man or woman (probably 20 beats fewer per minute than it is today). When you exercise, even full-tilt, your heart won't pound painfully because it will be moving your blood more easily through your cardiovascular system.

• An increase in lung efficiency and capacity. Your lungs won't have to work so hard to supply your body with the oxygen you need. Even when you exercise or do physical labor, you won't get out of breath so easily. You'll be able to do more without getting tired — like you did when you were in your 20s.

• An increase in blood volume. Your body will produce more blood plasma, hemoglobin, and red blood cells (oxygen "carriers") in its drive to become ever more efficient. Some studies show that a healthy man can increase his blood volume by as much as a quart through regular aerobic exercise.

• Better muscle tone and condition. Your body will look better, "tighter," as you change fat weight to lean weight.

• Lower blood pressure. Your vascular system will be improved as your blood vessels get stronger and increase in number in order to carry more oxygen throughout your body. As a result, your blood pressure will drop.

• Increased protection against disease. As you improve your body's efficiency, strengthen your heart and lungs, and improve your muscle tone, you'll be setting up a strong line of defense against a variety of diseases — not the least of which is heart disease.

The most important reason to exercise

Adding years to your life is not the only reason to exercise. In fact, it's not even the most important reason. The most important reason is that a program of regular aerobic exercise will vastly improve the quality of your life.

Now, this is a claim that can't be quantified — it's too subjective. But I defy you to find a man or woman who exercises regularly that does not believe that exercise enhances his or her life.

I know that exercise improves the quality of life because I used to be a couch potato. And now that I exercise on a daily basis, I know I feel better, stronger, and happier as a result. Plus, I've recommended aerobic exercise to thousands of my patients over the past two decades — and without exception, those who followed my recommendation reported that they felt better about themselves and the way they were living their lives.

The fact is that exercise makes us feel more astute, better about ourselves, and capable of achieving our dreams and goals. It makes us feel fully alive and in control of our own destinies. It also is one of the key, necessary elements of any plan to live to be 120 years old in good health. It's that simple.

How healthy is your heart?

Chances are you don't know what shape your heart is in. I can say that with a fair degree of confidence because most Americans don't.

Amazing, isn't it? Especially amazing when you consider that heart attacks will kill close to 1 million American men and women this year. And, yet, it's true. The vast majority — including those who are 35 years old or older and already among those most likely to experience what we commonly know as "heart trouble" — have never had even a resting electrocardiogram (EKG), let alone any of the more meaningful heart tests. Most people have no idea how good or bad a job their hearts are doing.

Well, prepare yourself, for as you continue your journey along the path to good health at age 100, you're going to become an avid student of your own heart. Before you begin your exercise program, you'll find out how healthy your heart is and you'll continue to monitor your heart's performance with regular checks.

Start with a "stress test"

Many fitness physicians recommend that every man or woman who is about to begin aerobic exercise undergo what is known as a "stress test" — a test in which a 12-lead electrocardiogram is used to measure the electrical activity of the heart while it's "stressed" by exercise. While a stress test is not necessary for every man or woman who is about to embark on a vigorous program of aerobic exercise, I do recommend it strongly because there is simply no safer or better way I know of to give your physician (and yourself) a true reading of your risk of heart attack or heart disease.

The typical stress test is administered to a patient as he walks or jogs on a treadmill, or pedals a stationary bicycle. More sophisticated tests make use of more advanced technology — monitoring the course of radioactive elements injected into the blood stream while the heart is under stress, for example.

Most often these tests — no matter what form they take — are used as diagnostic tools to detect early signs of heart disease before any changes can be detected in a regular or resting electrocardiogram. Additionally, stress tests are utilized by a few physicians, including Dr. Kenneth Cooper (at the Cooper Aerobics Institute in Texas) and myself to measure fitness levels.

The best way to measure risk

Dr. Cooper evaluated all the predictors used to evaluate more than 60,000 patients for heart attack risk. He found that measuring the amount of time a patient was able to work out on a treadmill was the most efficient and valid way to measure cardiovascular conditioning and to identify potential heart attack victims.

Over a 10-year period, I performed more than 5,000 exercise evaluations that included both stress tests and measurements of oxygen consumption. I found that the very best way to predict heart disease or attacks is to use the findings of a treadmill stress test in conjunction with a measurement of the patient's oxygen consumption divided by the heart rate. Though I added this new factor, my work still solidly validates Dr. Cooper's findings that a treadmill test is an extremely valuable tool — provided the test is conducted by a preventive medicine specialist who is willing to take the time to observe the person taking the test.

For some people, a "stress test" is a necessity

Though I recommend that everybody gets a stress test before starting to exercise, many people choose to skip the test, believing they are too young, too healthy — or that the cost is too high. I do, however, strongly urge and advise and caution you to get a stress test if you fall into any of the following categories:

• If you're a male over the age of 35 or a female over the age of 45 who is not physically fit. That is, if you score "fair" or below on the 12-Minute Test described on the following pages.

• If your immediate family history includes any individual who had heart disease before the age of 60.

• If you have any history of high blood pressure or diabetes — or if you have smoked within the past 10 years.

• If you have a known EKG abnormality or a history of any type of heart disease.

• If you have any history of chest pain, dizziness, or short-ness of breath — or if you have a family history of sudden death in a relative before the age of 40.

Remember, if any of the above circumstances applies to you, having a stress test is not an option — it's a requirement. This does not mean you won't be able to exercise aerobically to strengthen your heart. It does mean that your course of exercise may have to be moderated somewhat if — and only if — your stress test indicates a problem.

The 12-Minute Test

While the "gold standard" to determine your fitness to exercise is a stress test coupled with an oxygen consumption measurement, there is another way you can assess your level of conditioning — the so-called "12 Minute Test."

Originally designed by Dr. Kenneth Cooper, this test measures the distance you can walk, jog, or run in a dozen minutes, and gives a very accurate indication of your fitness level.

Quite simply, the 12-Minute Test measures your fitness by measuring your oxygen consumption. But it does it without fancy laboratory equipment and without the need to be hooked up to a machine. And, it is remarkably accurate. In one study, the 12-Minute Test was self-administered by 250 subjects. The results were then compared to results obtained by sophisticated treadmill tests under laboratory conditions — and the self-administered test results were right on the mark.

Here's how the test works

You can easily give yourself the 12-Minute Test. First, find or lay out a course two miles long. If you live near a high school or college, you may be able to use one of their indoor or outdoor tracks. Or perhaps you have access to an indoor track at a large YMCA or other club. If not, simply use the odometer in your car to measure a two-mile course in your neighborhood.

Then, dress comfortably, wear a watch with a second hand or an analog display so you can accurately gauge your time — and hit the course. Cover as much of that two-mile track as you can in 12 minutes. If you're able to run the entire distance, congratulations! You're in good shape. If not, run until you get short of breath, then walk until your breath returns to normal or near normal, and then run again. At the end of 12 minutes, measure the distance you managed to cover, using your car's odometer once again.

Use the chart below, a variation of a chart first developed and published by Dr. Cooper, to determine your physical fitness as measured by how much ground you were able to cover in the 12 minutes.

12-Minute Test

Men:

	Under 20	20-29	30-39	40-49	50-59	60+
Superior	> 1.87	> 1.77	> 1.70	> 1.66	> 1.59	> 1.56
Excellent	1.73-1.86	1.65-1.76	1.57-1.69	1.54-1.65	1.45-1.58	1.33-1.55
Good	1.57-1.72	1.50-1.64	1.46-1.56	1.40-1.53	1.31-1.44	1.21-1.32
Fair	1.38-1.56	1.32-1.49	1.31-1.45	1.25-1.39	1.17-1.30	1.03-1.20
Poor	1.30-1.37	1.22-1.31	1.18-1.30	1.14-1.24	1.03-1.16	.87-1.02
Very Poor	< 1.30	< 1.22	< 1.18	< 1.14	< 1.03	< .87

Women:

	Under 20	20-29	30-39	40-49	50-59	60+
Superior	> 1.52	> 1.46	> 1.40	> 1.35	> 1.31	> 1.19
Excellent	1.44-1.51	1.35-1.45	1.30-1.39	1.25-1.34	1.19-1.30	1.10-1.18
Good	1.30-1.43	1.23-1.34	1.19-1.29	1.12-1.24	1.06-1.18	.99-1.09
Fair	1.19-1.29	1.12-1.22	1.06-1.18	.99-1.11	.94-1.05	.87-.98
Poor	1.00-1.18	.96-1.11	.95-1.05	.88-.98	.84-.93	.78-.86
Very Poor	< 1.0	< .96	< .94	< .88	< .84	< .78

This is the beginning of your exercise program

If you score below "good," you fail the test. And, if you fail, you've got a lot of company. Most people — 75 percent or so — fail the 12-Minute Test the first time they take it. But, as soon as you begin to exercise, you'll quickly move from a "poor" or "very poor" score up the scale to "good," "excellent," and — ultimately — "superior"!

If, however, you are a male over 35 years of age or a female over the age of 45, and you score below the "fair" mark, please take a stress test — just to be safe.

The 12-Minute Test will not just show you where you are to-day — it will also show you the progress you are making as you put your exercise program to work in your life. It's a test you can administer to yourself whenever you wish — at no cost, and without any high-tech equipment. In fact, you can use the test itself as your aerobic exercise program when you start out — you can simply run/walk for 12 minutes a day, four or more times every week.

Before you decide to start with that, though, I want you to know exactly how much aerobic exercise I recommend, and I want you to be aware of the full "menu" of exercises that you can do — some of which will probably surprise you.

The difference between aerobic and anaerobic exercise

Your goal, as you exercise, is to achieve the maximum aerobic effect without crossing the line into "anaerobic" exercise.

If you remember, I define aerobic exercise as any activity that uses the large muscles of the body in a rhythmic fashion so that they deliver the oxygen the body needs to function well. With anaerobic exercise, on the other hand, the intensity of the activity is too high. The intensity is so high that the muscles are not able to deliver enough oxygen to meet the body's demands. As a result, we suffer what is known as oxygen debt. When this happens, lactic acid builds up in the muscles and we become fatigued. At the same time, anaerobic exercise can put undue strain on an unconditioned heart and put you at risk. Sports that involve intermittent high-intensity activity — basketball, tennis, racquetball, 100- to 400-yard sprinting, baseball, and football — are anaerobic.

Initially, only aerobic exercises are safe for those who are out-of-shape. These exercises include walking, swimming, bicycling, skating, jogging or running, jumping rope, certain types of dance and jazzercise, cross-country skiing, and rowing in a boat or on a machine. However, any anaerobic activity can be made aerobic if it is performed as a slower pace.

Because they cause sudden rises in blood pressure and heart rate, as well as the likelihood of oxygen debt, anaerobic activities should only be participated in by the physically fit. However, even professional, world-class athletes who earn their livings by participating in anaerobic sports also exercise aerobically. Many National Football League teams, for example, have developed jogging, dancing, or cycling programs for their players. They recognize the value of aerobics to build endurance. In fact, the best conditioned athletes are the aerobically trained long distance runners, swimmers, ballet dancers, cyclists, and cross country skiers.

Focus on cardiovascular endurance first

One of the basic effects of cardiovascular conditioning is to lower your pulse rate. When your pulse rate goes down, your heart will get more rest periods and will work less strenuously than the heart of the average individual who is not physically conditioned. For example, most long-distance runners (among the healthiest athletes) have a resting pulse rate in the 40 to 50 range. During normal activities like working or climbing stairs, these athletes typically have a pulse rate in the 60 to 70 range. Doesn't it make sense that an athlete performing a task with a pulse rate of just 70 is operating more efficiently than another individual performing the same activity with a pulse rate of 90 or more?

Typically, it takes about six weeks (if you are moderately fit) and about three months (if you are totally out of condition) for you to start to see and feel the results of your aerobic exercises. This is the reason I asked you to make a commitment to exercise for three months.

It is important for you to remember that there are many components to fitness, and that no one activity will give you everything you need. Complete physical fitness includes cardiovascular endurance, muscular endurance, strength, and flexibility. It will take time and work in a variety of different disciplines before you will be able to reach your full potential. For now, however, we will focus on your cardiovascular endurance — and the way to do that is to concentrate on aerobic exercise. In later chapters I'll teach you specific ways to improve your muscular endurance, strength, and flexibility.

Calculate your training heart rate

It is important to exercise properly. Simply starting a jogging or rowing program without a plan — and without a goal — is counterproductive. To establish a goal, you must first determine what is known as your "training" heart rate, or "THR." I have found that the best way to calculate this number is to subtract your age from 220 and multiply the result (your maximal heart rate) by:

- 60 percent during the first month of exercise,
- 70 percent during the second month of exercise, and
- 80 percent during the third month.

For example, if you're 49 years old, you would calculate your

THR by subtracting 49 (your age) from 220. That would give you a maximal heart rate of 171. Then:

- During your first month of exercise, multiply 171 by 60%.
  171 x .60 = 102 (your THR for the first month)
- During your second month of exercise, multiply 171 by 70%.
  171 x .70 = 120 (your THR for the second month)
- During your third month of exercise, multiply 171 by 80%.
  171 x .80 = 137 (your THR for the third month)

This number (your THR) is where your pulse rate should be when you exercise in order for you to get the maximum cardiovascular benefits without running any unnecessary risks.

Do not be concerned if you cannot maintain your exact THR when you exercise. Your goal should be to stay within 10 beats of this number. If you find that you cannot perform even minimal exercise for more than a few minutes without your pulse going way above your THR, it either means you are less conditioned than you thought, or that you have a primary lung, heart, or other physiologic condition that needs medical attention.

Don't push yourself

You may think your beginning THR is too low and, in fact, some individuals could start with higher rates. My experience has shown, however, that men or women who start with higher rates run the risk of injury without achieving fitness any more quickly. More important, most people who push themselves initially are the ones who quit — from boredom or, more likely, because they set unrealistic goals for themselves and give up rather than admit failure. So, use the THR prescribed for your age, using the formula above, and you'll find that exercise can be both beneficial and painless.

Remember that word "painless." It's important.

In fact, one thing that most of my cardiac patients notice, once they've been exercising for just a few weeks, is that they have not experienced the soreness that they expected when they started to exercise. They appreciate being able to achieve fitness without going through days when they're so sore they can't walk. I wish I could teach this lesson to directors of health spas who believe that pain is a necessary ingredient of physical conditioning. In my opinion, people experience muscle soreness only when they try to achieve goals they're not ready to achieve. It is for this reason that

I like to keep the THR on the low side and focus on this training rate rather than on an ultimate target.

Today, for example, I had a great workout. I ran four miles at a seven-and-a-half-minute-per-mile pace, then walked for two miles as I reflected on the day ahead, and then finished with a mile-and-a-half run at a nine-minute-per-mile pace. Workouts like this, when I don't push myself to the limit to see how hard I can make my body work, are my most memorable. Learn to enjoy your training and you will heighten your personal sense of well-being.

Learn to take your pulse

Having determined what your THR is, you need to know how to take your pulse. There are two places on the body where you can conveniently and easily do this: the radial artery at the wrist and the carotid artery at the neck.

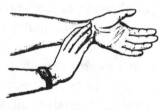

• *Radial artery pulse.* It is simpler and safer to measure your pulse rate at your wrist. To do so, place one hand in a relaxed, palm-up position. Then gently press the softest parts of the index and middle fingers of your other hand onto the base of the thumb (where your wrist bone joins your wrist). Do not press too hard, and don't try to get a reading with your thumb. You'll feel the pulse like a gentle drumbeat. Using a watch, count the number of beats you feel for 10 seconds. Multiply that number by six to get your pulse rate.

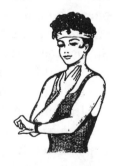

• *Carotid artery pulse.* If you can't find your radial pulse, try to find the pulse at the carotid artery in your neck. You'll find this pulse about two fingers below the angle of the jaw bone in front of the sternocleidomastoid muscle, which is the large muscle in the front of your neck (or just in front of that point). Again, use the pads of your index and middle fingers to feel it. When taking your pulse this way, it is extremely important not to press too hard or to make any sudden motions with your neck, or you might reduce the blood flow to your brain and become dizzy. Again, count the number of beats you feel in 10 seconds and then multiply by six to get your actual per-minute pulse rate.

If you can't find your radial or carotid pulse, ask a nurse, physician, or friend who has been trained in first aid to help you. Or, purchase a pulse watch, or other automatic device. If you do purchase one of these devices, make sure you get one that measures your pulse with a band that goes around your chest — not with a finger cot or an ear clip. Chest-band devices are much more accurate.

Keep a log

Once you master the technique, take your pulse each morning before getting out of bed (your resting heart rate) and record it in a log like the one below. Also keep track of your pulse rate at the beginning of each exercise session, at each session's mid-point (your training heart rate, or THR), and within five minutes following each session (your recovery heart rate).

Heart Rate Log

Date _____

Type of Exercise _____

Resting Heart Rate _____

Training Heart Rate _____

Recovery Heart Rate _____

• Your resting heart rate gives you an idea, first, of your current physical condition, since, as I said earlier, the lower an individual's resting heart rate, the better condition he or she is in. It also gives you a way to track your progress. Your heart rate will almost certainly be higher than the 40 to 60 beats per minute of a world-class athlete the first time you take it — but as you exercise aerobically, you'll see that number steadily decline.

In addition, your resting heart rate gives you a way to assess your stress level and to recognize overtraining (if it suddenly increases).

• Your training heart rate (THR) is your guide while you are exercising. If your heart rate is far above your THR, you are overexercising. If your heart rate is within 10 beats of your THR, you are exercising safely, without putting undue strain on your heart.

Your THR is a tool you can use to avoid unwanted anaerobic activity and to avoid muscle soreness.

• Your recovery heart rate, taken within five minutes of the end of your session, also lets you know if you are overexerting yourself. This rate should fall to 100 or below within five minutes. If it doesn't, either you've exercised too vigorously, or there is some other reason your pulse is too high. Take it easy. If your rate still doesn't drop after more moderate exercise, see your physician and explain the problem.

I strongly recommend that you maintain this log. It will help you to become aware of how much more efficient your body can be after just three months of aerobics. If, for example, you start with a resting heart rate of 90 and see it steadily decline over a period of three months until it's down to 75 or 80, you'll have proof in writing of one of the results of your exercise regimen. By being able to actually see the progress you've made in just a few months — knowing how much work you're saving your heart each and every day — you'll be much more likely to continue exercising for the rest of your healthy, long life.

Your log will also show you how you can lose valuable ground if you exercise for just a few weeks and then stop for a period of time before beginning to exercise again. Believe me, if you do interrupt your exercise program for even a short period of time, it will be reflected in your heart rate log.

As you become physically fit, after a period of several months, you'll discover that you no longer have to take your pulse to know whether you are exercising safely. You'll know — as all of us who exercise regularly do — when you are working out too strenuously. You'll have an inner feeling that tells you your cardiovascular system is being overtrained. If, however, you'd rather err on the side of safety, there's no reason for you not to continue checking your pulse rate regularly as you continue exercising. This is not only the safer course to follow, but will also enable you to keep on top of the headway you are making.

Stick with it

Of course, no amount of preparation or calculation will do any good unless you continue exercise once you begin.

Most people begin to exercise and then quit within four to six weeks. The most common reason they give is "boredom." That's why it's so important for you to find an activity you truly enjoy. One that you'll continue to enjoy over the long haul. Find the right exercise — walking, running or jogging, cycling, aerobic dance, cross-country skiing, or swimming — and then stick with it. If you enjoy more than one activity, alternate them weekly or from session to session. If you hate to exercise alone, find a partner — your spouse, a friend, your child, or even your dog. Many of my patients have enrolled in classes where they were able to mix socializing and exercising. Try step aerobics, slide aerobics, water aerobics — even martial arts like t'ai chi. Do whatever you have to do to make your exercise fun.

And be sure to exercise in moderation. You should be able to exercise, raising your heart rate to your own THR, with so little strain that you could carry on a conversation without gasping for breath — even in the middle of your session.

Here's the deal

If you do start your program, stick with it, and, at the end of three months, you do not notice a significant change in the way you feel and/or look — you can stop exercising. If, on the other hand, you do notice a significant change; if you've got more energy; if you look younger and more vital; then you have to renew your contract for another full year!

Of course, my ultimate goal is to convince you to exercise for your life — for the rest of your life. Right now, however, I'm not asking you for that kind of long-term commitment. Instead, I'm asking you to put into action the simple commitment you made way back in Chapter Four — to exercise according to my "Rule of 3s."

Simply stated, I want you to choose an aerobic exercise now and to participate in that exercise for 30 to 60 minutes, three times a week, for three months.

This is the least you can do

This is the least you can do to achieve positive results. And if you are completely out-of-shape, it may take you as long as three weeks before you can build up to the point where you can comfortably exercise for a full 30 minutes. Once you reach that stage, though, 30 minutes is your minimum.

You will need 10 minutes to "warm up" your cardiovascular system and reach your THR. No matter how fit you are, this will always be the case. Then, you must maintain your THR for at least 20 minutes. In this way, you will strengthen your heart muscle over time — slowly but surely. And always permit at least a 5- to 10-minute "cool down" after each exercise session.

Keep it slow and steady

I know a 57-year-old physician who, in 1970, at the age of 45, began a simple aerobic program of jogging for 30 minutes, three times a week. In 1975, when he had a stress test, he lasted 12 minutes on the treadmill. When he repeated the treadmill test in 1979, he lasted 15 minutes. In 1982, he went 19 minutes and 18 seconds. This represents an increase in his maximal oxygen utilization (the fuel of the muscles) from approximately 35 milliliters of oxygen per kilogram of body weight in 1975, to 61 milliliters of oxygen per kilogram of body weight in 1982. In terms of metabolic equivalents (METS), a medical term used to define energy requirements, it represents an increase in his maximal energy expenditure from 10 METS in 1975, to 17.4 METS in 1982. For the runner, this is equivalent to increasing his jogging speed from 5.9 miles per hour to 10.7 miles per hour — equivalent to going from running a mile in 10 minutes to running a mile in minus 6 minutes.

It may be hard to believe that slow, regular activity can make a 57-year-old male more fit than most men in their 20s, but that is exactly what it did in this case. This man's experience also confirms that it is not necessary to exercise every day, and that it is not necessary to spend hours and hours running, cycling, or swimming. If you perform your aerobic exercise regularly — following my "Rule of 3s," — you will have the same positive results. And if you miss one or two sessions each week, you'll feel yourself backsliding. It's that simple.

A word about weight training

At this point, let me make it clear that weight training — using one of the resistance machines like the Nautilus, or using free weights — will not and cannot take the place of aerobics. In order for you to exercise your heart muscle for maximum benefit, your exercise must be continuous and it must elevate your pulse rate to your THR for at least 20 minutes. This is not to say that you won't gain some aerobic benefits from weight training, only that the best way to improve your cardiovascular condition is through aerobics. The purpose of weight training is to develop strength — and I'll talk to you about that in Chapter Nine.

Your personal exercise prescription

Your personal aerobic exercise prescription is a combination of your mode of exercise (i.e., walking, cycling, etc.), plus your frequency (three days weekly), plus your intensity (the level needed for you to elevate your pulse rate to your THR). If you want to exercise more often than three times a week, I recommend that you change your mode on the extra exercise days so that you train different muscle groups. You could, for example, cycle three days and swim two, or alternate walking with rowing.

Don't think that "harder is better" as you progress. Many people think they're improving their routines on exercycles or rowing machines by increasing resistance. But increasing resistance places much more strain on your heart than increasing the frequency of arm or leg revolutions. A better approach would be to increase your pedal revolutions from 70 to 80 per minute, or your rowing strokes from 20 to 40 per minute.

Whenever you work too hard or too often, you risk injury. The most common exercise injuries are usually caused by breaking in a new piece of equipment like running shoes or a new bicycle, or by starting a new type of activity. Take it easy when you begin any new routine — and ignore the erroneous and dangerous concept of "no pain, no gain."

There are safe ways to ease into new forms of exercise. You can take courses, seek out health clubs where you can get instruction, hire a one-on-one trainer for a lesson or two, or join a cycling or running club that has a training course for beginners.

You have a lifetime to become physically conditioned — so take your time.

Warm up and cool down

Before you begin, learn the first rule of safe exercise: you have to warm up and cool down.

1. <u>Warm-up</u>. Any athlete knows that you don't just hurl your

body from rest into exercise. It's necessary to warm up first. I recommend the following easy warm-up before you start each session:

•   Do some stretching exercises for your arms, legs, and back. An ideal warm-up exercise is the "Sun Salutation" that I describe in detail in Chapter Ten.

•   Jog slowly in a circle for about 15 seconds, then walk for 15 seconds, jog again for 15 seconds, and walk for an additional 15 seconds.

2. <u>Cool-down</u>. While virtually everybody knows about the importance of a warm-up before you start to exercise, many people don't realize that it is equally important to cool down when you're done. If you jog or run, for example, several minutes of walking is the ideal cool-down. If you dance or use an exercise machine, slowly jog in place for a few minutes before you completely relax.

The fundamentals of successful aerobic exercise

Here's some more information that you need to guarantee productive, safe workouts.

1.   Choose an activity that you not only enjoy, but one that is suitable for your lifestyle.
2.   In the beginning, schedule your exercise sessions like regular appointments — and stick to your schedule until exercise becomes a habit.
3.   With aerobics, understand that total time spent exercising is more important than the distance traveled. It's more important to exercise continuously for 30 minutes than to run a quick two miles.
4.   Avoid running on a course that passes in front of your house — you might be tempted to quit your session early.
5.   Set a time for your jog or walk — say 40 minutes total, or 20 minutes away from your house and 20 minutes back. That way you won't have to worry about how much distance you're covering.
6.   If there is a wind blowing, start your exercise into the wind so that your return trip will be more comfortable.
7.   Drink plain water frequently while you're exercising — one or two 8- to 10-ounce glasses every 20 minutes, and at least that much before you begin. You don't need electrolyte

solutions or anything containing sugar — and keep in mind that cold water is absorbed more rapidly on warm or hot days.

8. If you live in a hot climate, avoid outdoor exercise when the humidity is high or you will dehydrate quickly. Instead, exercise in an air-conditioned mall, at a health spa, or in your own air-conditioned home.

9. Choose appropriate clothing. Wear layers of clothing in cold weather so you can remove the layers as you warm up. In hot weather, wear clothing that allows ventilation and perspiration to keep your body temperature low (nylon shorts or nylon and mesh singlets, for example). And always wear suitable, comfortable shoes.

10. Alternate days of hard exercise with days of easy exercise to avoid injury. If you cycle and go 40 miles one day, make the next day a rest day or a day on which you go for a shorter (20- or 25-mile) ride.

11. Take lessons whenever possible, especially if you've chosen to do something that requires skill such as swimming or cross-country skiing.

12. Walking is inexpensive, can be done anywhere, and requires no training. However, make sure your walks are brisk — walk about 3 or 4 miles per hour, or approximately 120 to 140 steps per minute. A brisk arm swing increases your energy needs and makes walking more vigorous.

13. If you use hand-held, 1- to 5-pound weights, you will increase the intensity of your walking workout even more. You must pump the weights as you walk, however — don't just hold them.

14. Never jog with hand weights. It will increase your risk of knee injury.

15. Jogging at a pace compatible with your THR is an excellent exercise. However, if you jog more than 30 miles a week, you run the risk of knee injury.

16. Hill work and track and speed play are the most common causes of injury in joggers.

17. Jogging does nothing to strengthen your upper body or your quadriceps muscles (those on the front of the thigh). To strengthen those muscles you may want to alternate jog-

ging with rowing or cycling.

18. Aerobic dance presents as much potential for injury as run-
     ning, especially if done more than three times a week. Proper
     conditioning for dance requires a mix of aerobics, muscu-
     lar strength, and flexibility — best done with the supervi-
     sion of a professional.

19. Swimming is an excellent aerobic activity. It offers low
     injury potential and a high degree of flexibility. Plus, it
     exercises both your upper and lower body muscles. Take
     lessons to learn to do the strokes correctly. Alternate be-
     tween a work stroke (like freestyle) and a rest stroke (like
     side stroke) so you will be able to swim for 30 consecutive
     minutes or more.

20. When you use a rowing machine, remember that it is better
     to work on increasing the frequency of your strokes than to
     increase resistance.

21. Cycling is an excellent aerobic exercise. However, whether
     you use an exercycle or a 10- or 12-speed bike, certain rules
     apply. To avoid injury and improve your conditioning, use
     spinning — a technique of pedaling between 70 and 100
     revolutions per minute. Use toe clips or specialized pedals
     to improve the efficiency of the exercise by making sure
     both the quadriceps and hamstring muscles are worked.
     Adjust your seat so there is a 15- to 20-degree bend in your
     knee when the pedal is at 6 o'clock (the bottom of the stroke).
     When pedaling, keep your knees in close and your heels
     flat.

22. Cross-country skiing is one of the most strenuous and most
     beneficial activities, because it exercises both your arms
     and legs vigorously. The popular machines that simulate
     the motions of cross-country skiing provide less strenuous
     exercise. This may be the best type of exercise for healthy
     people, but is too strenuous for those individuals with heart
     or lung problems.

Double your fitness level in three months

If you don't have heart disease, chronic lung disease, asthma,
or another degenerative disease, it should take you about three
months to reach a relatively good level of fitness. Even if you're

out-of-shape, I believe that you can double your fitness level in three months by exercising aerobically for 30 minutes a day at your THR for three days per week.

It is important for your three months of exercise to be consecutive — not split up by periods of inactivity. In other words, if you exercise for a month and then stop, you'll have to start your three-month commitment over again. Even the most fit individual loses ground if he or she stops exercising. And it takes just about six weeks of inactivity to set anyone back to square one.

Three months is, however, just your first goal. It will take nine to 12 months for exercise to become a positive habit. Even so, the first three months are crucial. During this time, you will learn that exercise is enjoyable — even as you begin to look and feel healthier.

By taking my challenge — by living up to your commitment to my "Rule of 3s" — you will find in yourself a new balance between mind, body, and spirit. You'll be so satisfied with the results after just three months that I know you'll never go back to a life that doesn't include aerobic exercise for a healthy heart and longevity.

In the next chapter, I'll teach you formal methods of stress management. Remember, however, that you don't need to progress with this next step until you feel ready. Meanwhile, the practice of aerobic exercise will, itself, help you to "defuse" the stresses in your life.

Actions to Take

• Start your program of aerobic exercise. Exercise for 30 minutes a day, three times a week, for three months. If you cannot perform aerobic activity because of some physical limitation, consider yoga or t'ai chi.

• Keep a heart rate log. Record your resting heart rate before you exercise, your training heart rate (THR) halfway through your sessions, and your recovery heart rate within five minutes after finishing.

• Don't quit. Be patient with yourself. Enjoy your exercise the way a 5-year-old enjoys his play.

Chapter Eight

Step 4:
The Balm of Tranquility

All of the Eastern medical systems stress the importance of a peaceful mind for total well-being. The Chinese express this as the state when one feels:

Refreshed, like swimming in the ocean,
Relaxed, like resting in a grassy meadow,
Growing, like the tallest evergreen,
Refined, like polished gold, and
Radiant, like a sunset.

Stress is deadly

Stress causes hypertension, the so-called "silent killer" that's a root cause of heart attack, stroke, and even kidney failure. Stress is a contributing factor in ulcers and has been pointed to as a possible cause for immune system weakness. Some research indicates that in a worst-case scenario — that is, if you're a so-called "hot reactor,"

and sudden stress causes a jolt of epinephrine to hit your heart —
stress can lead to sudden death.

Even if stress doesn't kill you, it can make your life miserable.
It can lead to blinding headaches, the feeling that your stomach is
tied in knots, and debilitating back pain. It can make you lash out
at loved ones and co-workers. Long-term stress causes mental an-
guish and can irreparably damage careers and relationships.

One study showed that a remarkable 85 percent of all visits to
primary care physicians are for stress-related illnesses. A second
study, a recent survey by Northwestern National Life Insurance of
Minneapolis, Minnesota, measured job-related stress and showed
that almost half the workers surveyed experienced job-related stress
in 1991 (the year of the survey). It showed that about 65 percent
had suffered exhaustion, anger, anxiety, or muscle pain due to stress,
and that 72 percent experienced three or more stress-related illnesses in the year prior to the survey.

The most common disease of our age

Stress is, according to many experts, the most common disease
of our age. Millions of men and women complain of feeling
"stressed out" by their jobs, by family pressures, or simply by life
in a world seemingly filled with stressors. These are the men and
women who shake their fists and curse at other drivers on the
crowded interstate, who scream at co-workers over slight misun-
derstandings, who sit silently at their desks being eaten alive by
their own unresolved anger — and who die red-faced and gasping
because they couldn't find a parking space.

I always feel a sense of sadness and frustration when I see people
being literally robbed of life by stress. I don't feel sorry for them
because they're faced with so-called "stressful" situations. Stress,
after all, is a part of everyone's life. But, my heart goes out to them
because I know from experience how easy it is to deal with stress
in a positive way. How easy it is for anyone to safely manage any
stressful situation.

Stress management has to be learned

However, stress management must be learned. It's not something that comes naturally to most people. That's why so many
medical centers, corporations, large and small businesses, organi-

zations, and professional groups sponsor stress management classes or seminars. And that's why I decided to make stress management an integral part of my seven steps to a century of great health.

During the past 20 years, I have helped thousands of patients cope with stress and have spoken to hundreds of professional groups about stress management. I have met with stressed executives, managers, physicians, dentists, and others. Through this, I have gained insights into what causes stress, how to manage stress — and even how to use some stress in positive ways. In this chapter, I will share my insights with you as the fourth step in my seven-step program. First, however, we need to clearly define stress.

Know the enemy

Physical stress is easy to understand. If you run up three flights of stairs, the physical stress on your body is immediate and easy to recognize. Depending on the shape you're in, that exercise could cause a slight burning in your thigh muscles — or it could make your leg muscles ache and knot, your heart pound, and your chest heave as you gasp for breath.

Your body's reaction to sudden emotional stress is also immediate and easy to recognize. If, for example, you're driving along a road late at night and a deer leaps in front of your car, your body will react instantly. As you slam on the brakes, your mouth will go dry, your pulse will quicken, and your breathing will become ragged.

Other forms of stress are less obvious. You can, for example, experience some stress if you have to make a difficult decision and spend days, or even weeks, agonizing over a course of action that might have serious consequences. You might experience great stress if you're working on a major project for a difficult boss — laboring under the knowledge that your performance could literally make or break your career. Even preparations for a happy event can create stress — the marriage of your daughter, a long-delayed European vacation, the purchase of the 36-foot sloop you always wanted.

In every case, stress is related to an event or chain of events. It doesn't appear from nowhere. Stress is always a reaction to what we call a "stressor."

There's no such thing as a stress-free life

You can't eliminate all the stressors in your life. Deer are going to leap in front of your car. You're going to have to deal with difficult employers, employees, and relatives. You're going to have to make difficult business decisions and personal decisions. And there are some stressors that you wouldn't want to eliminate even if you could — cheering your son through a championship soccer game, for example, or having to make a speech after you've won the Nobel Prize!

Though you can't eliminate stressors from your life, you can change the way you react to them. Just as you can physically condition yourself to run up three flights of stairs without physical stress, so can you mentally condition yourself to deal with the stressful situations in your life.

The bottom line is that since you can't control the stressors in your life — whatever they might be — you must learn to control your reactions to them.

As the comic strip character Pogo said, "We have met the enemy, and he is us!"

I first became convinced of this after reading the works of Dr. Hans Seyle, considered the "father of practical psychology."

The destructive power of stress

Dr. Seyle, in his book *Stress Without Distress*, defines stress as "wear and tear" on the body caused when the human organism (the body and mind as a whole) responds psychologically and physiologically to different demands. Anything — pleasant or unpleasant — that disturbs the equilibrium (sense of balance) of the body or the mind can be defined as a stressor.

Humans, Seyle goes on to say, experience stress either positively or negatively. If stressors or stress events lead us to destructive reactions, the stress must be viewed as negative. If, on the other hand, stressors lead us to constructive reactions, the stress itself may be viewed as positive. Stress, then, in and of itself, is neither positive nor negative. It is our reactions to stress that are positive or negative.

If we react negatively to the stress in our lives over the long term — if we continually have destructive reactions to stressful situations — the stress itself begins to wear at and tear down our bodies the same way that long-term abuse will ultimately destroy a piece of machinery. The physiological effects of this long-term wear-and-tear can include common colds, substance abuse, cancer, nervous breakdowns, ulcers, heart attacks, and, eventually, death.

For a "hot reactor," stress can be deadly

It is even possible for a negative reaction to stress to lead to sudden death, if the individual under stress is what we call a "hot reactor." In a hot reactor, the wear-and-tear phenomenon makes itself known as a sudden jolt of the hormone adrenaline — a jolt so strong that it literally destroys the heart muscle. Medical science once thought the cause of death in these cases was heart attack, but it is now widely accepted that stress itself was the cause.

There are hot reactors who are "type A" personalities — hard-driving executive types who never take the time to relax, who eat too much of the wrong food, who smoke and drink, and who appear to be, even at first glance, ideal candidates for sudden death due to stress. Then there are hot reactors who are "type B" personalities — easy going, laid-back, seemingly always in control. What makes an individual a "hot reactor" has nothing to do with his personality. It has to do with the way his body reacts physiologically to stress. His blood pressure will jump without any symptoms of heart disease, and his cardiac output (the amount of blood that flows from the heart) will drop — thus making the ultimate stress-related heart injury possible.

The good news for hot reactors is that they can protect themselves by using stress management techniques and by taking prescribed medication, if that is indicated.

A personal experience convinced me

The "hot reactor" was first clinically described by Robert Elliot, M.D., and I must admit that when I first read about Dr. Elliot's research I was skeptical. But then, in 1984, I had an experience with a 42-year-old male who died suddenly. Prior to his death, this patient was, by all accounts, in good health. He had some problems that seemed to be associated with a decision he had made in 1983 to start his own business, but those problems were minor. He gained weight, he had more head colds than usual, he developed a skin rash, and he found himself getting irritable with his children and losing interest in family affairs. He had a normal insurance physical in 1983 and a normal general physical in early 1984. Both of those exams disclosed no heart anomalies. And yet, late that year, he was found dead in his kitchen, where he'd gone to prepare breakfast.

An autopsy showed that while the blood vessels leading to his heart were normal, the damage that had been done to his heart muscle was the type of damage usually associated with the sudden blockage of an artery. This is exactly what research done by Elliot and others has shown is the result of a sudden stress-related jolt of adrenaline in the body.

All the news about stress is not bad

Some stress is actually good. For example, the stress that you feel when you need to do well on a job assignment can give you the added energy you need to achieve your goal.

And, by learning stress management, you can turn a would-be negative into a positive. By learning to deal with your stress, you will become a stronger person. You will be more resilient. You will interact with your spouse and your children in positive ways. You will begin to work better and to be more productive. You will enjoy your leisure time more fully, loving the moment and not fretting about either the past or the future. All because you learned how to deal with stress in positive ways.

Stress is a personal matter

Before you can begin to change the way you react to stress — by turning destructive, negative reactions into positive, constructive reactions — you must first identify the things in your own life that produce stress.

It seems that this should be easy, but it's not. There's no set formula here. Something that creates stress for one man or woman may not be stressful — and may even be pleasant — to another. In fact, studies conducted several years ago to test the stress-adaptability of test pilots working for the U.S. Department of Defense showed just how personal this matter truly is.

In these tests, it was discovered that pilots were actually comfortable in situations in which they were in great danger — at times when the average person would expect to be paralyzed by fear. Many of these same pilots, though, hit uncomfortable stress levels when faced with some situations that many of us deal with comfortably on a day-to-day basis — like a room full of preschoolers. Everyone has a different "comfort zone."

In their book, *The C Zone*, researchers Robert Kriegel, M.D. and Marilyn Kriegel, M.D. say that there is a "comfort zone" (C zone) wherein each individual is comfortable with the amount of stress he or she is experiencing, as opposed to a "zone of distress" wherein the same individual is uncomfortable. And they say that these zones are different for each individual when faced with the same stressful situations. In other words, a situation that is well within your comfort zone could subject someone else to unbearable stress — and you might not be able to handle a situation that that person would find comfortably challenging.

Some people, for example, find that speaking in public is an exhilarating experience. The natural stress associated with the experience of delivering a speech in public is experienced by these individuals as a positive, and they perform better because of it. Other men and women are simply terrified at the prospect of public speaking. They have a negative, destructive reaction to this stress and may experience nausea, memory lapses, or worse if forced to perform before strangers.

Recognize your body's signals

Because of the personal nature of stress, I obviously can't give you a list of specific things that will cause you stress and then tell you how to deal with each of those in turn. I can, however, teach you about what I call the root causes of stress and about stress-generators in general. And I can explain how you can begin to recognize your own stressors.

Most of us know when we are experiencing stress, though we may not recognize it by that name. But we know we're experiencing something that makes us uncomfortable or uneasy. That's because our physiology undergoes changes when we're faced with a stressful situation. Like all members of the animal kingdom, when you are placed in a situation that you perceive to be dangerous or fearful, your body reacts immediately, pushing you to choose between "fight or flight."

According to researchers, here are just a few of the things that happen as your body prepares to take action:

• Your adrenal glands start to pump out adrenaline. This "rush" makes your heart beat faster and harder and elevates your blood pressure.

• Cortisone is also secreted by your adrenal glands to shut down the parasympathetic nervous system that would otherwise calm the "fight or flight" response. However, because this glandular secretion is part of your body's immune system, over-secretion in times of stress can lead to a reduction of your normal resistance to infection. Over-secretion of cortisone can also reduce your stomach's resistance to acid and lead to ulcers.

• Your thyroid gland starts to secrete a hormone that speeds up your metabolism. However, if this metabolic increase continues, nervousness and insomnia can be the end result.

• The amount of sugar in your blood rises to give you a burst of energy. In response, your pancreas starts to produce insulin to balance the sugar. Overworking your pancreas, however, can lead to diabetes — or, at the very least, to low blood sugar (hypoglycemia).

• Your liver starts to pump out cholesterol to provide your body with fuel, and your platelets start to get "sticky" and ready to plug up a wound. Over time, however, elevated levels of cholesterol and thickened blood will begin to adhere to blood vessel walls, and potentially lead to heart attack and stroke.

The easiest way for you to determine that you're experiencing stress is to pay attention to your body's signals and learn to recognize when you're in this "fight or flight" mode, so you can do something about it before the stress starts to wear and tear at your body.

Stress signals sent by your body may include dry throat, headache, upset stomach, pain in the neck or lower back, heart palpitations, and rapid breathing. Signs and signals of longer-term stress include shortness of temper, a lack of interest in hobbies and pastimes you typically enjoy, a lack of the desire to spend time with your family members or loved ones, sleeplessness, a lack of sexual desire, the loss of appetite, and fatigue in the morning.

Learn that you have alternatives

Obviously, there are some truly dangerous situations that you might have to face in which physically fighting or fleeing are, literally, your only options. If, for example, you're confronted by an armed robber, your body will get you geared up to fight or run for your life. However, in most stressful situations, when our bodies are telling us to either bolt or do battle, neither of these options is truly appropriate. Instead, we react by either flying into a rage (fighting) or by internalizing our fear and anger — doing damage to ourselves in the process.

One of the purposes of stress management is to teach you alternative ways to react to that stress, so that when you acknowledge the signals being sent to you by your body, you don't have to vent your anger or internalize it.

First, though, you need to identify the root causes of your stress. This will enable you to determine just how to go about managing the stress they trigger.

Stress is caused by conflict

In general, stress originates with some sort of conflict. This conflict disturbs the equilibrium of the mind or body and leads to the imbalance that Seyle identified. That imbalance leads to stress. The greater the conflict, the greater the imbalance — and, ultimately, the greater the stress.

Your stress may stem from a conflict with another person, or from a conflict with the rules of an impersonal organization or institution. You may also have an inner conflict — if your actions are not in agreement with your values or true beliefs. If you're not living your life the way you want to or in a way that you find admirable or worthwhile.

In stress management we don't focus on the situation. That's not the problem that we try to solve. Instead, we focus on how to deal with the stress that's generated by the conflict. And, we do this by teaching you how to control your reactions to stressful situations — how to turn a negative, destructive reaction into one that is positive.

Changing the way you look at it

Perhaps you're stressed because you have a demanding boss who wants everything done his way — even though you completely disagree with him. No matter how hard you try, he makes you feel threatened and afraid of losing your job.

What if you are able to accept the fact that your demanding

boss may not know as much as you do about some things, but he's still your boss. And since he signs your paycheck, he has a right to demand that you do things his way. Once you realize that you can't change him, you might decide that your best course of action is to agree, and simply earn that paycheck. Wouldn't that de-stress your interaction with your boss?

Now imagine that you are able to view the loss of your job not as a financial disaster, but as an opportunity to find a better job and to grow and possibly make more money. Wouldn't that eliminate the negative stress in this situation?

Perhaps you've suddenly lost your job. You're overwhelmed by self doubt and the hassles and worry that go with trying to find a new job. The result? Immediate stress.

Or perhaps you're stressed because you are working from dawn to dusk, day after day, forced by your need to succeed or to make money into spending too much time at the office — when you'd rather spend that time with your family. Not only are you in conflict with yourself here (you're not doing what you really want to do), but your stress may be compounded because you're afraid you're losing your family's love.

In this situation, you need to be able to analyze your decision to work 80 hours a week and recognize that the root cause of your stress is the conflict between your values (the importance of your family) and your actions. Once you understand why you're stressed, you'll be able to take action to do something about it. You might choose to switch to a less-demanding job — or at least cut back on your hours. Alternatively, you might choose to continue putting in the long hours, but do it for a positive return — to do something good for your family by earning extra money. Whatever your course of action, you would be able to eliminate the negative stress by eliminating that conflict between your beliefs and your actions — by changing the way you look at the situation.

You have to take charge

The fact of the matter is that the primary cause of negative stress in our lives is the conflict created by our own perceptions, values, and beliefs. That means that each of us has the power to control our own reactions to stress and to determine if those reactions will have a positive or negative effect on us.

This is why, in the several hundred stress management talks I've given to professional groups over the years and in my work teaching my patients how to use the tools of stress management, one of the first things I do is to drive home the point that we each have to "own" our own problems. You are not stressed by "him" or by "that thing" or by "those events." You are stressed by *your reactions* to them. You have to take responsibility for your own stress by admitting that your reactions are the problem.

By "owning" your own problems, you empower yourself to stop fighting the people or institutions (the situations) that are your stress-triggers. By doing that, you get to save energy you would otherwise expend trying (unsuccessfully, I must add) to change those people, institutions, or situations. You can't change the unchangeable, so save your energy for actions that can really help you.

Set your priorities

Once you've taken the responsibility for dealing with your own stress, you need to have a clear understanding of what's really important to you before you can take action to eliminate the conflicts in your life.

Start by making a list of your priorities. Relax with your eyes closed for a few moments. Then, open your eyes and list the things that are important to you, in descending order of importance. Your list (which should be updated every three months, because priorities do change over time) might look something like this:

> GOD
> FAMILY
> > Wife
> > Children
> > Parents
> > In-Laws
>
> WORK
> > Career goals
> > Job relationships
> > Current projects
>
> HEALTH
> > Staying well
> > Fighting disease
>
> MONEY
> > Managing on a daily basis
> > Investment objectives
>
> RELATIONSHIPS

Then, after relaxing for a few more moments, answer the following questions:

- What do I most like to do?
- What do I least like to do?
- What do I wish I could do that I don't or won't do?
- What qualities do I admire most in other people?
- What qualities do I dislike in others?

This simple self-examination will give you a good idea of what your priorities are. By concentrating on these priorities, you'll be able to identify the root cause of the stress generated by a specific situation. Then you'll be able to defuse the stress by understanding how you need to change your perception of that situation in order to get rid of the conflict.

The "Rule of 3s" as applied to stress management

Any form of stress management that you use will make you healthier and happier. You'll be healthier because you'll be intervening in or stopping the wear-and-tear process that leads to so much illness. And you'll be happier because you'll feel better and you'll no longer be reacting inappropriately to the conflicts in your life. You'll no longer be causing rifts between yourself and your loved ones. Instead, your actions and your beliefs will be in harmony. You will be living a life that is truly worthwhile.

But, you'll need some specific techniques to effectively manage all of the different kinds of stress in your life. So, use another one of my "Rule of 3s" as your guide to the three different types of techniques that you need to master — one step at a time.

1. Learn some sort of relaxation therapy.
2. Learn an intervention technique that uses your sense of touch, sight, smell, or hearing to relieve acute tension.
3. Use some form of physical activity to dissipate the destructive effects of elevated levels of hormones on your body.

1. Relaxation therapy

You should practice some form of relaxation therapy every day. The specific technique that you choose is, of course, a matter of your personal choice.

My personal favorite is Transcendental Meditation (TM) — a technique that allows your mind and body to achieve a settled, relaxed state that is more restful than sleep.

However, TM is not something that you can learn to do by reading a book. You need to take formal instruction. At some point, you may wish to take that step. For now, though, I'll teach you an alternative form of meditation that is very effective for stress management. I call this form of meditation "focus meditation." By this I mean that you relax by focusing your mind on an image, a sound, a word — anything that allows mind-body stress reduction.

Focus meditation, step-by-step

Here, then, is a step-by-step description of the technique I have taught many of my patients with no prior experience in meditation:

1. Look at a clock to check your starting time. You should keep your session to between 10 and 20 minutes.
2. Sit in a chair or on the floor, in any way that's comfortable for you.
3. Close your eyes.
4. Allow thoughts to enter your mind unbidden. Do not try to prevent thoughts. Do not try to "force" specific thoughts. If you want to think about something that enters your mind, you can — or you can just let it go and allow the next thought to enter.
5. After one to three minutes, gently open your eyes for 10 to 30 seconds.
6. Close your eyes again.
7. Let your thoughts flow. If you have pleasant thoughts, that's fine. If your thoughts are troubled, don't fight them. Keep your eyes closed and your mind open for one to three minutes.
8. Open your eyes for about 30 seconds.
9. Close your eyes and concentrate on a pleasant image or place you know of or can imagine. Or repeat a calming word or phrase over and over and over again in your mind. Some people use words like "peace" or phrases such as "I am more relaxed" or "I feel calm" or even a prayer like "I love the Lord." If thoughts enter your mind, allow them to come in. But as soon as it's comfortable, reintroduce the phrase or image that you were focusing on before.
10. Continue to meditate for 10 to 20 minutes. Don't worry about the time. You can open one eye to glance briefly at a

clock without interrupting your meditative state.

11. When the 10 to 20 minutes have passed, gently stretch, and then slowly open your eyes.

12. Sit quietly for a minute or two before resuming your regular activities with renewed energy. If, as some people report, you feel slightly fatigued when you finish your meditation, simply close your eyes for a few more minutes to relieve that fatigue and let energy flow through your body.

A few words of advice

Do not try to meditate in bed or in a completely dark room. You don't want to confuse meditation with sleep. And never meditate after meals or after a period of strenuous exercise. The best time to meditate is before you get started in the morning, or before dinner at the end of your workday. Meditate at least 90 minutes before bedtime, because meditation will give you energy and might make sleep difficult.

Perhaps most important is for you not to become compulsive about meditation. Enjoy it. While the most beneficial way to meditate is once in the morning and once in the evening, it has been shown that regularity is more important than the amount of time spent. In other words, it's better to meditate once a day for 15 minutes each and every day, than to randomly meditate twice in one day for 20 or 30 minutes.

Hundreds of thousands of people meditate each day, and the results they describe (the same results I've experienced from my own practice of TM for about 20 minutes each morning and evening) are remarkable. In fact, many of my patients routinely thank me for enlightening them about meditation and say it's the single item in my program that has had the most profound impact on their lives.

The benefits of meditation

Meditation obviously guards against hypertension. But that's not all. In 1978, physiologist R. Keith Wallace, a researcher at the University of California in Los Angeles, discovered that even novices experienced profound relaxation and significant changes in breathing, heartbeat, and blood pressure.

Wallace also proved that, with the long-term practice of TM, blood pressure, near-point vision, and hearing (three of the so-called "markers" of aging) all improved. In fact, his research showed that meditators who had been practicing TM for less than five years had a biological age five years younger than their chronological age — and those who had practiced TM for more than five years had an average biological age 12 years younger than their chronological age. In addition, he discovered that meditators visited doctors and entered hospitals only half as often as those in a control group, and that they experienced 80 percent less heart disease and more than 50 percent less cancer than those in the control group.

Some people avoid Transcendental Meditation or other forms of relaxation therapy because they have the mistaken idea that these practices are "religious" and may go against their own beliefs, whatever those might be.

To be sure, in some cultures, meditation is part of the practice of religion (in Zen Buddhism, for example). However, just as not all religions include the formal practice of meditation, not all meditation is religious. To put your mind at ease about this point, note that when you meditate, you can focus on any phrase or image. You don't have to concentrate on something with a religious connection in order to achieve a relaxed state.

2. Acute intervention techniques

In addition to the regular daily practice of some form of relaxation therapy, you need a technique that you can use to intervene (step in) during times of heightened stress. Obviously, you can't stop in the middle of a business meeting that's going badly, or in the middle of an argument with your spouse to take time out for 10 minutes of meditation. So, you need to know what to do when you realize that you're under acute stress. You need to have a way to relieve that tension.

One of the best ways to release tension is to laugh. Many people — including me — find that something as simple and silly as a child's wind-up toy gives them the laugh break they need when they are stressed out.

Now, you can't always meditate and you can't always pull a wind-up toy from your pocket or purse. But there are things you can do that have the same end result.

The secret here is to use your senses — sight, touch, hearing, taste, or smell — to calm you down. For example, perhaps you have a favorite painting, or a piece of music you love. Visualize that painting or listen to that melody in your head for a moment, and let your mind wander, recalling a relaxed, happy time.

This type of acute intervention technique is an excellent way to dissipate the physical effects of stress — even in the middle of a business meeting. It works because it is very difficult to feel worry, fear, anger, or resentment when you're visualizing pleasant sights and sounds. By taking a brief moment to tune out and calm down, you will be able to re-focus on the important issues that you have to deal with.

Long term, the regular practice of this sensory form of stress intervention will help raise your stress threshold. In other words, it will take more stress to push you to the point where you're feeling angry or fearful.

3. Hormonal stress reduction

Earlier in this chapter, I explained how stress triggers the release of certain hormones in your body — and how the elevated levels of these hormones can be destructive. The purpose of hormonal stress reduction is to dissipate these destructive forces through some form of physical activity.

This is the ultimate stress management technique. The importance of lowering these elevated hormonal levels through exercise can't be overstated. In fact, all the relaxation therapy in the world, coupled with acute intervention, is much, much less effective if it is not coupled with hormonal stress reduction. Though any type of activity will work, the best activity for this purpose is some form of aerobic exercise, whereby the pulse rate is elevated to a predetermined level. So, if you've already started the aerobics program that I outlined in the last chapter, you've already begun to practice this stress management technique.

The benefits of aerobic exercise go far beyond hormonal stress reduction. Aerobic exercise lowers your blood pressure and your heart rate. It lowers your body fat and increases your muscle mass and efficiency. It lowers the level of serum epinephrine in your blood, if it is chronically elevated. And it raises the level of your endorphins (the hormones that have been identified as the body's "natural opiates"), causing what is commonly known as "runner's high" — the sense of extended well-being that is reported by some runners during and after a training session.

By the way, you need to be aware that there is currently a debate as to whether this endorphin release is a positive or negative, since too much of this hormone may lessen a runner's ability to feel good without a high endorphin level. That has not been my experience, nor has it been reported by my patients and friends who exercise aerobically. However, as is the case with continuing research on antioxidants, keep your eyes open for new research information about endorphins.

In any case, the benefits of aerobic exercise far, far outweigh any possible negatives. In addition to the benefits I already mentioned, as you exercise and your heart, lungs, and circulatory systems improve, nutrients and oxygen will move more easily to all parts of your body, wastes will be more easily removed, your enzyme system will be in better balance, so your muscles will relax more completely. You'll sleep better, your endurance will increase — and you'll have fun.

In the next chapter, I will teach you how to exercise using either free weights or resistance machines, to strengthen your muscles and your bones. Meanwhile, as always, remember to be patient with yourself. Don't take the next step until you're ready.

Actions to Take

• Take the self-test on pages 113-114 every three months to clarify the things that are really important to you and establish your priorities.

• Use the results of that test to help you find the root causes of the conflict in any stressful situation, and train yourself to change your perceptions to eliminate the conflict.

• Learn and practice the following stress management techniques on a regular basis:
1. a form of relaxation therapy, such as Transcendental Meditation,
2. an acute intervention technique, and
3. a form of physical activity — preferably aerobics, yoga, or t'ai chi to reduce hormonal stress.

Chapter Nine

Step 5:
The Yang of Strength

Oriental wisdom holds that everything in the universe is divided into "yin" and "yang," and that a balance must be maintained between these two elements. When we apply the yin/yang principle to exercise, we balance the yang energy of weight training (for strength) with the yin energy of stretching exercises (for flexibility).

Use it or lose it

Well-conditioned muscle cells, the kind of cells you had when you were an active young boy or girl, can contract about half of their resting length and support more than 1,000 times their own weight. But, if you don't exercise, this ability diminishes as you age — starting at about age 30. By the time you're 65, you will have lost from 30 to 40 percent of your strength and about 12 percent of your muscle mass. By age 75, if you continue your sedentary life, you could be among the 25 percent of American men or

65 percent of women who are unable to lift any object weighing more than 10 pounds.

In other words, when it comes to your muscles, it's a clear case of "use it or lose it!" And the earlier you start to "use it" — by getting involved in a weight training program of your own choosing — the better off you are.

Now, I'm not recommending a weight lifting program that will get you ready to enter a Mr. (or Ms.) Universe contest. I am talking about a sensible weight training program — one suited to your age — that will work together with your aerobics training to keep you fit and healthy as you age.

The benefits of weight training

I was pleased when the American College of Sports Medicine (ACSM), a professional organization of exercise experts of which I am a fellow, recently changed its "official prescription" for good health to include (for the first time ever) sessions of "moderate intensity" weight training with barbells, weight-bearing calisthenics, or resistance training machines. According to the ACSM, such a routine is a necessary part of any health program either for overall fitness or for a more active and agile old age.

Scientific evidence and my own experience with my patients has proved to me, beyond any shadow of a doubt, the many benefits of weight training programs.

A major defense against aging

First and foremost, weight training is a major defense against premature aging. You must have strength in order to remain active as you age. Weight training permits you to go rock climbing instead of playing shuffleboard. It allows you to run in a marathon instead of playing checkers.

Weight training increases your muscle mass — and the more muscle mass you have, the stronger you are.

Muscle mass is built by the repeated contractions of muscle fibers against medium to high weight resistance. In terms of physiology, this depletes the muscle enzymes and breaks down muscle fibers. When the muscle fibers rebuild themselves, they rebuild stronger. In other words, the simple action of putting your muscles to work lifting moderate weights makes your muscles increase in size. And this happens no matter how old you are when you start. Weight training even helps ward off senility, according to a study at Scripps College in Claremont, California. That study showed that men and women who exercise regularly perform better than sedentary people in reasoning, reaction times, and memory tests.

But that's just the beginning — just the first benefit you will derive from your own strength training program.

Less fat without dieting

As your muscle mass increases, your metabolic rate speeds up, and that means you burn extra calories. Your body does this naturally, because muscle requires more calories than fat to sustain itself.

Lean muscle mass consumes energy 24 hours a day, just to sustain itself. And pound-for-pound, muscle burns from 40 to 50 more calories per day than fat. So, if you replace just five pounds of fat with five pounds of lean muscle, you'll burn off an additional 200 to 250 calories per day — even while you're sleeping.

This means that once you start weight training, you'll be able to eat more without gaining unwanted pounds — or that you'll be able to shed pounds without having to cut way back on your caloric intake. If you make weight training part of a total program that also includes aerobics and healthy eating (as I recommend), fat will seem to drop off your body, and the muscle mass that you've lost over the years will begin to reappear. Those embarrassing underarm "wattles" will be replaced by firm tissue. Your sagging chest will lift and shape.

A decreased risk of disease

Another benefit of increased muscle mass is that it decreases your risk of diabetes. As the muscle mass in your body increases, your body needs less insulin to get sugar, or glucose, out of your blood and into your tissues, where it's required for energy. This means that your body is less likely to experience a shortage of insulin, making it less likely that you'll develop what's commonly called "adult-onset" diabetes.

Weight training increases the ratio of so-called "good" HDL-cholesterol to "bad" LDL-cholesterol — and that means a reduced risk of heart disease. In addition, the body's muscles are its main reservoirs for protein, used by the body whenever you are sick, injured, under stress, or recovering from surgery. The stronger your muscles, the more protein you'll have available for your body in these times of heightened need.

Arthritis pain relief

According to a study conducted by scientists at Tufts University, weight training may even help lessen the pain of both rheumatoid and progressive osteoarthritis. While the scientific jury is still out on this claim, apparently the "burn" — a comfortable warm feeling in the muscles that accompanies weight training — lessens the discomfort associated with arthritis. At the same time, weight training strengthens the muscles, tendons, and ligaments around joints, easing joint-stress and, hence, easing arthritis-associated pain.

Bone strength

Perhaps the most important benefit of weight training, however, is its ability to add bone density and actually replace bone cells that have been lost as part of the aging process.

According to very recent research, bones and connective tissues react much the same way that muscles do when challenged by weights or resistance — they grow stronger. This is important because bone weakness can lead to seemingly spontaneous fractures — the kind that occur when an older man or woman breaks a hip simply by stepping off a curb. And too many out-of-shape senior citizens sustain fractures by stumbling, tripping, or falling while walking. These may seem like minor problems until you stop to think that fractures are the leading cause of hospitalization for older Americans.

Bone strength is particularly important for older post-menopausal women who find themselves facing osteoporosis.

An integral part of my seven-step program

For all these reasons — plus the fact that strength training makes you feel healthier, stronger, and much more in control of your life — I advise all my patients who are physically able (and that's virtually everyone) to get involved in weight training along with aerobics and a healthy diet. And that's why I made weight training an integral part of my seven steps to a century of great health.

Speedy results

One of the great things about weight training is that it has nearly immediate results. You won't achieve anything like your full potential right away, to be sure. But you will, within just a few short weeks, notice changes in your body and in the way you feel and act — no matter how old you are when you start. In fact, I guarantee you'll start feeling stronger within two weeks, and that within three months, you'll double, or maybe even triple, your strength. My guarantee is backed by research.

One study focused on a group of 90-year-old women in Boston's Hebrew Rehabilitation Center for the Aged. This study showed that the women — involved in a weight training program for just eight weeks — almost tripled their strength and added significantly to their muscle mass.

Another study — this one at Tufts University's research center on aging — tracked a dozen men aged 60 to 72 as they took part in a training program using a machine designed to strengthen leg muscles. After just three months of three sessions weekly, the muscle mass in the men's legs had increased significantly. Their extensor muscles (those that straighten the knee) were, on average, 107 percent stronger. And strength in their flexor muscles (those that bend the joint) were, on average, 226 percent stronger.

Researchers at McMaster University in Ontario proved that upper body strength can be quickly increased when they enrolled 14 men aged 60 to 70 in a 12-week program. The men exercised only one arm. When the study ended, lifting strength in the trained arms had increased an average of 48 percent, while strength in the untrained arms remained unchanged.

In terms of the real world, not the laboratory world, this means that with weight training you'll be able to carry a heavy potted plant without breathing hard. You'll be able to reach to the highest shelf in your closet and lift down that box of books you haven't seen in five years. You'll be able to play with your grand-kids (or great-grand-kids) without getting worn out. You'll win more tennis matches and drive tee shots closer to the green. You'll have more energy for work, for play, for sex — for the business and pleasure of everyday living.

Tailor your program to suit yourself

The days when weight training meant making three weekly trips to a dank, dark gym where some heavyweight in a black t-shirt would put you through your paces using barbells and dumbbells are long gone. These days, you can work out at home, using a variety of machines or "free weights" (barbells and dumbbells). Or you can join one of the new generation of gyms where trained professionals will help you exercise using the very latest in strength-training equipment.

No matter how busy you are, you can fit weight training into your schedule. In fact, if you follow my recommendation — namely to exercise the major muscle groups in moderation at least twice weekly and preferably three times weekly — you'll spend only one to two hours a week exercising (including warm-up and cool-down). Refer to Appendix B and Appendix C for complete outlines of my beginner and intermediate weight training programs.

You can easily tailor a weight training program to meet your schedule, your budget, and your personal taste.

A program based on moderation

As I noted earlier, weight training goes by many names, including resistance training and strength training. The scientific name for this process is "isotonic training." That's just a fancy way of saying that the process involves making specific muscles in different parts of your body work harder than usual by pitting them against a resistance — the weight. The more weight you can lift or push, the more resistance you can overcome. Over time, the muscles doing the lifting or pushing and overcoming the weight resistance become bigger. That is, they increase in mass.

When many people think of weight training or strength training, they immediately imagine themselves grimacing and straining — looking like the overbuilt heavyweight lifters at the Olympics struggling to raise hundreds of pounds over their heads.

Nothing could be further from the truth. The weight training I advocate and urge you to do on a regular basis involves regular, moderate challenging of the major muscle groups in your body. Please note the word "moderate" in that sentence. That means lifting moderate weights (weights heavy enough to require exertion, but light enough so that you can lift them eight, 10, or 12 times in succession) according to a reasonable schedule (two or three times weekly).

Learn the jargon

Some knowledge of weight training jargon is necessary as you follow a weight training program. Each time you lift a given weight in a given exercise, that is called a "repetition." A group of repetitions ("reps") is known as a "set." A typical routine might include three sets of 10 repetitions. In other words, you would perform the motion of the exercise 10 times, then rest for a brief period, perform another set of 10 reps, rest again, and then perform another 10-repetition set.

The "pyramid technique" of lifting (which should be used only by advanced, properly trained weight lifters) involves increasing the amount of weight you lift with each set and decreasing the number of reps. For example, you could lift 100 pounds 12 times in one set, increase the weight to 120 pounds and decrease the number of reps to 10 in the second set, then increase the weight you lift to 140 pounds and decrease the number of reps to eight in the third set.

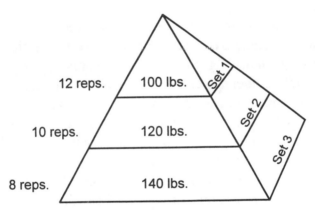

A "super set" is another technique that should be used only by advanced weight lifters. In this technique, opposed or non-related muscle groups are exercised without resting between sets. For example, you might work opposing muscles by doing a biceps exercise and then immediately follow that with an exercise that works the triceps on the same arm, without resting between sets. Or you might perform a chest exercise and then a leg exercise, again without resting.

There are basically three types of weight training exercises you can choose from: strength calisthenics, free weights, or resistance machines. I discuss each of these in greater detail later in this chapter.

Technique is as important as weight

The building of muscular strength requires a process of tearing down and rebuilding muscle fiber. During the act of weight lifting, the muscle enzymes — the chemicals that allow for contraction — are depleted and replenished.

Most people who exercise — and most weight trainers — devote altogether too much time and energy focusing solely on the amount of weight being lifted. While there is no denying that the amount of weight you lift plays a major role in determining the results of your exercise, your form (lifting technique) is of major importance, since the proper form insures the best results and helps prevent injuries.

Over the decades, I have demonstrated to athletic trainers that I can teach people how to benefit from weight lifting if they maintain their form, rest between sets, and allow muscle groups to recover.

Schedule your sessions to let your muscles rest

A good rule of thumb is to rest 48 hours between sessions exercising any major muscle group. In other words, if you exercise your chest and shoulder muscles on Monday, you should wait until Wednesday before exercising that muscle group again. I have found that the most efficient system for the beginner is to work out Monday, Wednesday, and Friday utilizing all muscle groups. The intermediate lifter may choose to exercise four or even five times weekly, but even then should allow major muscle groups to rest and recover between sessions through the use of a "split" routine. With a four-day split routine, the chest, shoulders, and triceps would be exercised two days (Monday and Thursday, for example) — and the legs, back, and biceps would be exercised two of the other days (Tuesday and Friday, for example). This is outlined in Appendix B and Appendix C.

The time you spend resting between individual sets allows your muscle enzymes to replenish and permits you to lift a weight again and again without damage. In your initial training, rest periods of 30 to 90 seconds will be sufficient. As you advance in your training, and as the amount of weight you lift in each exercise increases, however, longer rest periods — about 2 or 3 minutes — will allow you to become stronger, build more muscle mass, and prevent the injuries that can occur with heavier weights.

Conventional wisdom has it that sets of 10 to 20 repetitions are ideal to train for muscle endurance, while sets of six to 10 reps should be used to build strength. Lifting any weight more than 20 times or less than six times provides little in the way of benefits, and a lot in terms of injury potential. (In advanced weight training, this "rule" is sometimes violated — but only for specific training goals.)

The value of "negative" work

One of the most important aspects of weight lifting or strength training also happens to be one that is overlooked by many trainers, and that is the value of what is usually called "negative" work.

When you lift a weight, that action is referred to as the "positive" aspect of lifting. Letting the weight down, or returning the weight to its starting position, is generally referred to as the "negative" aspect of lifting. In the 1970s, Arthur Jones — the founder of Nautilus — recognized the importance of negative work and designed his cam-operated weight machine to make full use of it. He proved that full utilization of negative work in weight lifting actually breaks down more muscle tissue, hence promoting more muscle repair and more build-up of both strength and mass. It not only promotes the building of strength and muscle mass, but also restricts injuries.

To fully utilize the negative aspect, he devised what has come to be called the "Nautilus Cadence" in lifting. Exercisers who use this cadence lift weights to a "1 - 2" count, then pause for a few seconds, and then return the weight to its starting position, slowly and under control, to a "1 - 2 - 3 - 4" count. Though the Nautilus Cadence was originally designed for use by lifters on the Nautilus resistance-type exercise machine, it is now widely used by weight lifters around the world. The Nautilus Cadence can be heard in gyms from New York to Tokyo.

Negative work is so important that there is even an advanced technique that has been developed in which a "spotter" helps the exerciser lift the weight (do the positive work), while the lifter himself controls the negative aspect of the exercise (lets the weight down or returns it to its starting position) without assistance. This technique, which has tremendous injury potential, is for advanced weight lifters only. It is best performed on a Nautilus machine or other device where the weights are easy to control. It can be dangerous when done with free weights.

Build your strength with calisthenics

One of the oldest and easiest forms of exercise — calisthenics — enables you to build your strength by using your muscles to overcome the resistance provided by your own body's weight. Indeed, many people start their weight training by doing nothing more complicated than exercises like bent-knee sit-ups, chin-ups, knee bends, leg lunges, and good, old-fashioned push-ups. See Appendix A for illustrations.

The push-up is an ideal example of how calisthenics provide weight training. When doing a push-up, you lift your body right from the floor. In other words, you overcome the physical force of gravity that's pulling you toward the floor. You overcome your body's natural resistance to being lifted. Each time you lift and overcome that resistance, you strengthen major muscles in your arms, chest, shoulders, and back.

Let me say now that I think calisthenics are an excellent form of exercise. In fact, I make one calisthenic exercise (bent-knee sit-ups) a continuing part of every exercise program that I recommend. However, there are two drawbacks to calisthenics, and, that's why I don't recommend that you do calisthenics as your only form of body strengthening.

First, if you are older, or if you've allowed your body to really deteriorate, you may find it impossible to do calisthenics — particularly chin-ups and push-ups, where you're required to overcome the substantial weight of your body.

And, if you are in good enough shape to do calisthenics, you will quickly reach the point where the exercises lose much of their effectiveness. You will strengthen your muscles so fast that you will need to do an ever-increasing number of each exercise to derive any benefits, or you will need to add external weights (a back pack, for example, if you're doing sit-ups).

Moving on to harder exercises

How do you know when an exercise is not giving you the benefits you want? That's easy — as soon as the exercise becomes too easy.

In other words, as soon as you have strengthened a muscle or a group of muscles enough that you are able to do sets of 10 or 12 repetitions without resting for more than a few seconds between each set — it's time to make the exercise more difficult. You need to work your muscles to the point where they feel almost exhausted after each set of repetitions. If you don't feel that "exhaustion," you're not benefiting from the exercise.

You can see, then, that with calisthenics, you will constantly have to challenge yourself by adding external weights or by increasing the number of reps you do in each set. Sooner or later, you'll be doing 100 push-ups with your partner sitting on your back, or 50 chin-ups with frozen turkeys strapped to each ankle.

Start off the right way

While calisthenics are fine in the beginning, you'll soon want to move on to more sophisticated and efficient forms of exercise. So, I recommend that you start the right way — with a program that involves calisthenics plus some sort of weight or resistance equipment.

Strength-building equipment

There are two basic kinds of strength-training equipment:
1. Free weights
   - barbells — long bars with weights at each end
   - dumbbells — weight-carrying bars short enough to be grasped by one hand
2. Resistance machines (sometimes called "multi-station gyms" because they give you the ability to get a full-body workout by changing resistance loads and exercise stations)
   - the standard weight/stack pulley arrangement, with which you increase or decrease resistance by adding or removing weights which are then pulled or pushed using bars and a system of pulleys
   - rubber cable systems, which use a variety of adjusting devices to increase or decrease resistance
   - shock absorber systems, which also use various devices to adjust resistance

There are, as you might imagine, positives and negatives associated with any system.

Free weight systems

Free weight systems offer low cost and convenience. You can set up your gym in almost any room in the house and work out when you wish, wearing whatever you wish. All you need to get started is a barbell with a set of weight plates, at least two dumb-bells, and a bench.

Starting weight sets can be purchased inexpensively. Benches vary in price according to their degree of sophistication. At the very least, you want a bench that has a wide, stable base that won't wobble. Make sure it's welded at the joints, not just bolted to-gether — and make sure the padded bench is comfortable. Also check to make sure the uprights (the U-shaped holders that support the barbell off the bench) are wide and strong. You should be able to obtain a complete free-weight set for $200 to $1,000.

Drawbacks to free weights include the need for a "spotter" — someone to help you if you get into trouble using too much weight — and the danger that you might drop a weight on your toe or some other body part during exercise.

Resistance machines

Machines offer safety along with the convenience of being able to work out at home — provided you have enough room that you can set aside for a permanent work station. Your best bet for a resistance machine is an all-in-one machine — that is, one that can be changed into varying configurations to exercise different parts of your body.

The downside to resistance machines is that they're expensive. The typical all-in-one machine retails for about $700, and some cost several times more than that.

Don't buy a machine until you're ready

My recommendation is that you ultimately work out using one of the resistance machines, but that you start with a combination of free weights and calisthenics. Why? Because it doesn't make a great deal of sense to spend $1,000 or so on a resistance machine until you are positive that you're going to put it to work. Once you have the "exercise habit," start to look for a resistance machine you like.

I'm not going to recommend a specific machine, because that's a choice that must be made by you personally. Research these machines — their capabilities and their costs — by visiting a local gym and talking to people who use different machines. Write to manufacturers for literature and visit retailers who sell a variety of exercise machines to do some comparison shopping. Make sure you actually climb aboard any machine you're thinking of purchasing, either in the showroom or at a gym.

Understand your workout

Before looking at specific exercises or exercise programs, it is important to understand exactly what it is that you're trying to accomplish as you work out.

As I explained earlier, you strengthen your body by making specific muscles in your body work harder and increase in mass and strength by pitting them against some form of resistance. It is impossible, however, to isolate individual muscles in the body when you work out. For that reason, weight training or strength training concentrates on exercising major groups of muscles that work together. The groups of muscles you should concentrate on in your exercise are the back, chest, shoulders, abdominal, biceps (the "front" of your upper arms), triceps (the "back" of your upper arms), and legs.

How much you lift depends on you

In weight training, the object is not to lift as much as you can lift. The object is to lift what you can comfortably lift a dozen times or so, in order to challenge your muscle groups. The amount that will be lifted by each individual, then, will vary. Some men and women will find it impossible to lift their own weight — and some won't be able to lift 10 pounds or even five. Others will be able to do chin-ups with ease and raise 100 pounds over their heads without breaking a sweat.

I recommend that you start light with every exercise, and then increase the weight you lift in small increments. Experiment. Try an exercise with just two-pound dumbbells — or five pounds or 10. If it's too easy, increase the weight by as little as possible until you find the weight you can lift eight times, but no more.

If you are able to raise a 100-pound barbell over your head one time, you'll find that for exercise purposes, your ideal work-out weight will be about 50 percent of that amount — or about 50 pounds. If you can do one squat with 50 pounds on your shoulders, your work-out weight will be about 25 pounds.

Warm up first

When you exercise, you stretch not just your muscles but the ligaments and tendons in your body as well. Like a cold rubber band, a tendon or ligament is likely to snap when suddenly stretched. For this reason, it is important that you warm up, slowly stretching and getting your body ready for work, before you actually start to exercise. I recommend, as a warm-up, the same regimen I recommended for your pre-aerobic warm-up, namely:

1. Do some stretching exercises for your arms, legs, and back. An ideal exercise is the "Sun Salutation" that I'll describe in detail in the next chapter.
2. Walk for five minutes on a treadmill or ride an exercycle. If you don't have either of those machines, jog slowly in a circle for about 15 seconds, then walk for 15 seconds, jog again for 15 seconds, and walk for an additional 15 seconds. Repeat this cycle for about five minutes.

Cool-down and recovery

You also need to give yourself a cool-down period. I recommend an easy stretching session and some easy jogging or walking for about five minutes following your weight-training exercise. This will help you to avoid strain and injury.

Remember that you need to allow yourself sufficient recovery time between your exercise sessions. As you exercise, you'll be working muscle groups by forcing them to overcome resistance repeatedly until you reach a point where each group can't comfortably lift any more. That's quite a work out! If you do this every day, you'll overtax your muscles and risk injury.

Meanwhile, experience has shown that the best and fastest way to stimulate muscle growth — increase your strength and turn flab into lean muscle — is to exercise your major muscle groups and then to allow yourself a recovery period of at least 36 hours (preferably 48 hours).

Remember, though, that your lean muscle will be burning calories while you rest, so, even in your recovery period, you are becoming more fit, healthier, leaner, and meaner.

The importance of timing and breathing

However you choose to exercise, it is important that you take your time. Allow about two seconds to lift a weight (count "1 - 2") and four seconds when you lower it (count "1 -2 - 3 - 4"). Rest between each set for about one minute. Make sure you breathe properly. Exhale when you lift the weight or strain against resistance — inhale as you relax or lower the weight.

Now, let's get down to work!

While it is not within the scope of this book to set up training programs that will meet every exerciser's specific needs, I have attempted to set up complete programs for both beginner and intermediate level weight lifters. (See Appendix A for detailed instructions and illustrations of each exercise, and Appendix B and Appendix C for a complete outline of my beginner and intermediate programs.) Advanced lifters have enough experience and awareness of the vast amount of research material available to set up their own programs.

Tips for successful weight training

- During the first six weeks of your exercise program, concentrate on form. Make sure you know how to do each exercise properly in order to get the maximum benefits and to avoid injury. Don't worry about weight levels. After you know how to do each exercise, increase weights incrementally.

- As you move from beginner to intermediate weight lifting programs, you can and should seek advice on how to do specific exercises from a personal trainer. Other exercisers will be more than happy to help you out, but their advice may lead you astray and could cause injury. Get help from a professional.

- Work out regularly. Set a schedule and stick to it as much as possible. The ideal for beginners, again, is three times weekly. Do this for three months, and I guarantee you'll be overjoyed with the results.

- Keep a training record. Record how much you're lifting, how many reps you're doing, etc. This is necessary if you're going to add resistance incrementally. Being able to track your own progress will also keep you involved and interested.

- Stay with it! Skipping an occasional work-out is okay. If you quit for a month or more, however, you'll be right back where you started.
- There are additional pieces of weight lifting equipment you can buy — gloves, weight straps, and weight belts, for example. All have advantages and disadvantages. As you progress in your own program and become familiar with these accessories, you will be able to decide for yourself if they would be helpful to you.

The rewards of weight training

A weight training program is not to be taken lightly. (I intended that pun — honestly I did!) In the beginning, take it easy. Don't overdo it. Ideally, you can set up a balanced program between free weights and resistance-type equipment. In this way, you'll exercise all your muscles without any duplication of effort.

And remember, just as regular meditation has cumulative effects that go far beyond the benefits derived from just one session, regular exercise will have a cumulative effect on every area of your life. The least you can expect is better health and increased strength at age 100 and even beyond.

In the next chapter, I'll tell you about specific ways you can avoid and treat back pain or back injury.

Actions to Take

- Score a "passing" grade on the 12-Minute Test (see Chapter Seven) before beginning weight training. If you are over 40 or have a history of heart or back trouble, get your physician's okay before you start. You'll be able to exercise — but you may need to tailor your program to meet your specific needs.
- Decide what kind of weight training program you're going to do, and when and where you're going to do it.
- Do it!

Chapter Ten

Step 6:
The Yin of Flexibility

When we balance the yang of weight training with the yin of stretching exercises, a major benefit — in terms of Western medicine — is that it protects us from back injury. And back pain — no matter what its cause — can be debilitating. When you suffer from back pain, you're unable to do the things you want to do. You can't dance, or play, or exercise, or make love — or do much of anything at all with full enjoyment. It can make strong young men and women whimper like babies. And it's common. It is estimated that up to 95 percent of the population has suffered from lower back pain at least once. And if it only happened once to most people, they'd be thrilled. Unfortunately, in many cases, back pain becomes a chronic condition.

Back pain is a serious problem. Statistics show that back pain accounts for 93 million sick days annually, or about 40 percent of all job absenteeism. It is second only to upper respiratory infection when it comes to causing "sick days" — and those days are taken off at a huge cost in terms of lost productivity and profits.

Your back is a remarkable machine

Chances are excellent that you don't even think about your back until it hurts. That's because it's a remarkably put-together machine that enables you to bend and turn and twist and lift. The primary component of this machine is your spine, which houses your spinal cord and the nerve branches that run off that cord. It also houses about 2,000 muscles and thousands more ligaments. Your spine itself is comprised of 24 bones (vertebrae) that are separated by shock absorbers known as discs, the sacrum (the bone that attaches your spine to your pelvis), and the coccyx (tailbone).

The spine is, indeed, a remarkable machine, able to function beautifully, until ...

Well ... until you age.

As you age, the bones in your spine mature. In your mid-20s, degeneration begins. More bone cells are destroyed than your body can replace. At the same time, your spinal discs — those little shock absorbers between the vertebrae — start to lose water content and harden. The muscles in the abdomen and lower back that keep your spine properly erect and curved also begin to weaken, most often as a result of either misuse or disuse. And therein lies the cause of most back pain.

Some back pain is caused by disease

To be sure, some back pain is caused by disease. Scoliosis, a condition typically diagnosed in preadolescent girls whose spines curve abnormally to the side, for example, can lead to extreme back pain if the misalignment is centered in the lower spine (lumbar region). Hyperlordosis or "swayback" can also cause low back pain, as can cancer (in rare cases), degenerative arthritis, sciatica, osteoporosis, and other diseases with tongue-twisting Latin names.

However, if you suffer from back pain, it's very likely that your pain is not an indication of scoliosis or osteoporosis, or, in fact, any disease — other than the disease that comes with what might be called a "normal" aching back. That's because only about 10 percent of all back pain is caused by disease.

Most back pain is caused by strain

Your back pain is probably the result of straining the muscles or ligaments in your lower back — because of an injury or because of simple overuse. The most common cause of back pain, in fact, is an injury caused by a simple action, like lifting a heavy suitcase the wrong way, twisting suddenly while picking up a package, or bending over too far to retrieve a dropped pencil.

Other common causes of back pain stem from disuse (like sitting for extended periods of time in front of a computer), strain on the muscles of the lower back during pregnancy, bad posture, or stress.

Since the vast majority of back pain is not caused by an underlying illness, curing that pain is relatively easy. And prevention is as simple as spending a few minutes exercising each day.

Curing back pain

If you do have an episode of back pain — and you know it's because of an injury or strain — what should you do? Here's the course of action I recommend to my patients.

1. As an initial treatment, consider going to a chiropractor for manipulation.
2. Rest in bed for a day or two, avoiding bending, twisting, or lifting as much as possible. The best way to rest is on your side or back with your knees drawn up. This reduces strain on your muscles, ligaments, and discs.
3. Apply ice for the first 24 hours. Use a regular ice pack, or dump some cubes in a plastic bag. In a pinch, use a bag of frozen carrots (another good use for this yellow vegetable). Wrap the ice in a thin towel or a cloth napkin and place it directly on the painful area. The ice will not only reduce pain, but it will also reduce swelling and mitigate any muscle damage. I recommend applying the ice for about five minutes, three to four times a day.
4. If possible, have somebody massage the ice on your back for five minutes. This technique is even more effective at reducing pain and swelling than the simple application of an ice pack.
5. After the first 24 hours, replace the ice treatments with moist heat treatments. If you can lower yourself into a tub of hot water, do so. It's the best way to apply moist heat. If not,

use an electric heating pad together with a water-soaked
sponge-wrap or damp, hot towels.

6. If you can, take an anti-inflammatory such as buffered as-
    pirin or an aspirin substitute (Ibuprofen) every four hours.

7. Try herbal remedies including burdock, horsetail, slippery
    elm, and white willow bark. You should be able to find
    these at a health food store. If the pain is severe, talk to
    your family physician, who might prescribe muscle relax-
    ants. But I recommend this only if you're in dire need,
    since drugs can be addictive and can cause unpleasant side
    effects — including depression. In other words, treat your
    back pain as naturally as possible.

8. Don't stay in bed too long. After two days, start moving
    around the house. Over the next several days, go for short
    walks. When you're relatively comfortable walking, start
    to do some mild stretching exercises to increase your flex-
    ibility. Within two or three weeks, you should have re-
    turned to normal and be able to comfortably do what you'd
    normally do.

9. Once you're back to normal, start exercising to avoid re-
    current problems. It's easier than you think.

A word of caution

Since some back pain is disease-related, see a physician you
trust without delay if:

•   You suffer from severe back pain that doesn't respond to
    rest, heat, and anti-inflammatory medications such as
    aspirin or Tylenol.

•   You experience symptoms of weakness or numbness in your
    hands and feet.

•   You have pain from your neck radiating down your arm,
    or back pain radiating down your leg.

•   If there's no improvement, even in very minor pain, in a
    week or so.

•   If you experience other symptoms, including bladder or
    bowel problems, in association with back pain.

Prevent recurring problems with calisthenics

If, like millions of Americans, you suffer from recurring back pain — the kind that never really goes away — and flares up from time to time — you need to improve the strength and flexibility of your hamstrings, stomach muscles, and the muscles of your lower back when it's extended (straight) and when it's flexed (bent). These muscles and ligaments act like the "guy wires" that support radio or television antennas, or the lines that support the masts on a sailboat. They allow flexibility with strength.

Exercise, quite simply, must be your number one backache prevention strategy. This means exercising daily, if you already have a back problem, and three times a week for prevention. Here are a few exercises you can easily do to prevent back injuries or pain by strengthening your spinal supports:

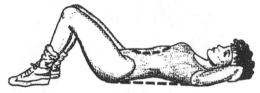

• *Pelvic tilt.* Lie on your back with your knees bent and your feet flat on the floor. Using your abdominal muscles, pull in your stomach while you tilt your hips upward, flattening your lower back against the floor. Hold this position for 10 seconds and then relax. Repeat 10 times.

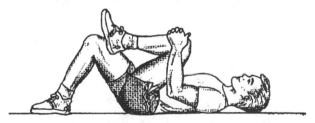

• *Single knee-to-chest stretch.* Lie on your back with your knees bent. Pull one knee into your chest until you feel a comfortable stretch in your lower back and buttocks. Hold for 10 to 15 seconds. Repeat with opposite knee. Repeat 2 to 5 times.

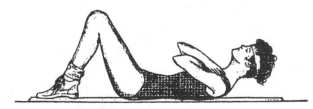

• *Bent-knee sit-up.* Lie on the floor with your arms folded across your chest, your knees bent, and your lower back pressed to the floor. Lift your head and shoulders slightly off the floor toward your knees and hold for 10 seconds. Repeat 10 times.

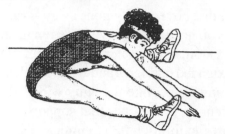

• *Sit-and-reach.* Sit on the floor with your legs stretched and your feet spread apart. Reach forward with your hands toward your feet as far as possible, and slowly return. Do not bounce when trying to reach for your feet. The motion should be smooth.

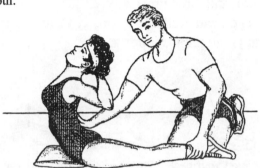

• *Hyperextension back exercise.* Lie on your stomach with a cushion under your abdomen. Clasp your hands behind your head while your partner holds down your feet and lower back. Now lift your body at the waist and hold for a few seconds.

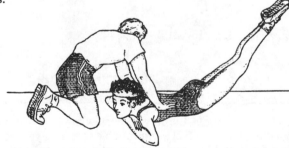

• *Hip lift.* Lie on your stomach with your arms crossed under your chin while your partner holds down your upper body. Lift your legs as far as you can and hold for a few seconds.

• *Angry cat stretch.* Get on your hands and knees with your back level. Slowly arch your back, lowering your head and pulling in your stomach muscles. Hold for 2 seconds and return to starting position. Repeat 5 to 10 times.

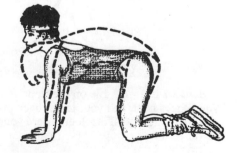

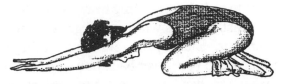

• *Mid-back stretch.* Kneel on the floor, extending your arms and torso forward, and sitting back on your heels. Reach out as far as you can, keeping your head down. Hold for 10 seconds. Repeat 3 times.

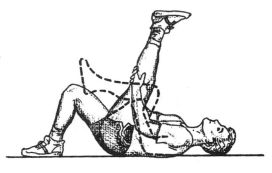

• *Hamstring stretch.* Lie on your back with your legs bent. Pull one leg in toward your chest, supporting the back of your thigh behind your knee. Attempt to straighten your knee until you feel a comfortable stretch on the back of your thigh. Hold for 10 to 15 seconds. Repeat with opposite leg. Repeat 2 to 5 times.

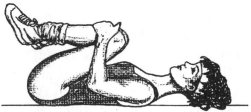

• *Double knee-to-chest stretch.* Lie on your back with your knees bent. Pull both knees into your chest until you feel a comfortable stretch in your lower back. Hold for 10 to 15 seconds. Repeat 2 to 5 times.

Add lower body exercises to your weight training program

In addition to calisthenics, you need to include exercises in your weight training program that strengthen your lower body. The best exercises for this are squats (knee-bends) and stiff-legged deadlifts. (See Appendix A.) If you have a history of back pain, avoid leg curls and leg extensions, since these put stress on your lower back. I also advise you to avoid standing barbell biceps curls, because if you use too much weight, you'll have a tendency to arch your back for extra lifting power, putting excessive stress on your lower back.

Use common sense to avoid injury

In addition to strengthening your back with exercise, there are precautions you can take to avoid injury or strain in your everyday life.

- If you have to pick up something heavy, don't bend forward from the waist and hips with your legs straight. Instead, bend your knees and rely on your stronger thigh muscles.
- Lift smart. Keep you lower back bowed in — not hunched out — when you bend over. Keep the object that you're lifting as close to your body as possible, and never twist or jerk with something heavy in your arms. If you must turn, turn with your feet — not your upper body.
- Don't sit for long periods of time. Get up. Take a break. Stretch. Massage your tight muscles.
- If you have to sit for long periods of time while working, make sure your chair supports your spine — particularly the lumbar area or lower spine — and that it fits your body and supports your thighs. Keep your feet flat on the floor with your legs bent at 90 degrees.
- Invest in a back pillow for support. There are several different types on the market, so you'll have to experiment to find the right one for you. One option is an inflatable pillow that you can take with you wherever you go. Simply inflate it until it's floppy (not rigid) and place it behind the small of your back when you're at work, in a car, or on an airplane. A good inflatable pillow can be ordered from Medic-Air Corp. of America, 16 N. Chatsworth Ave., Larchmont, NY 10538.
- If you do computer work, your screen should be 14 to 16 inches away from your eyes to avoid glare and neck strain. Set your screen at eye level, directly in front of you — not off to the side.
- If you spend a lot of time on the telephone, invest in headphones. Cradling the receiver with your shoulder leads to neck pain.
- If you're stuck in a seat for a long time — on a transatlantic flight, for example — exercise in your seat:
  1. Lift your knees alternately toward the opposite elbow, while reaching slightly toward the knee with your elbow. Repeat 15 times with each knee.
  2. Bend forward slowly in your seat until your chest touches your thighs. Then gently return to an upright position. Repeat about 20 times.

Both of these exercises will stretch the spine and prevent stiffness. They should be repeated every two hours you spend trapped in your seat.

- If you have a beer-belly, exercise to get rid of it. All that excess weight can push your spine out of alignment.
- If you smoke, quit. Research shows that smoking may reduce the blood flow to the vertebrae which protect the disks and, hence, lead to lower back problems. (See Special Supplement I at the end of this book for help.)
- Reduce stress in your life following the advice I gave you in Chapter Eight.

How about sex?

Contrary to what you might think, sex is not harmful when you've got a bad back (provided you don't make love in positions that add injury to injury). It can actually be therapeutic since lovemaking reduces tension and exercises the lower back. The trick here is to make sure you're comfortable. Verbalize. Let your partner know exactly what feels good for you and what causes pain. But ...

- Avoid positions that require you to arch your lower back so that your spine is bowed forward, toward your belly. Assuming a "swaybacked" position like this puts a great deal of pressure on the posterior portion of the spine (the back of the spine) and can lead to discomfort.
- Don't bend forward with your knees straight — even if you're lying down. Bending forward slightly is okay, provided your knees are slightly bent.
- Don't lie flat on your stomach or back with your legs straight. These positions flex the muscles that run from the front of the spine to below the hip joint and put too much forward pressure on the lumbar region of the spine. It's better to lie on your side with your knees slightly bent — or on your back with pillows or other supports under your knees.

Lest you think that following this advice leaves you no choices in love-making, here are a few positions that can afford pleasure without aggravating an already painful back.

- Both partners lie on their sides, with the woman's back to the man for rear entry. This is the best position if either (or both) partners are suffering acute back pain.

- If the woman is suffering back pain, she could lie on her back with her torso supported by pillows while her lover kneels to support her thighs with his thighs and arms.

- Another good position for a woman with back pain is to kneel astride the man, leaning forward slightly and supporting the weight of her torso on her hands. The same position, with the man's torso raised by a pillow or pillows and his knees bent and supported, is good for a man with back pain. (Avoid vigorously raising the pelvic area, though.)

- A kneeling rear entry position is good for a man suffering back pain, provided he supports his upper torso on his hands or arms and keeps his back slightly flexed (like a stretching cat). This is not a good position for a woman with back pain if she is too active or if her partner puts too much weight on her back.

In the final analysis, pleasurable (and therapeutic) love-making is possible even with back pain. And the extra care and consideration you and your partner show for each other during these times may even pay off with extra dividends as you discover new areas of sensitivity. Experiment and communicate. But don't feel you have to put your sex life on hold.

Yoga and your back

While many modern scientists and physicians search for new ways to treat back pain and new methods of preventing its recurrence, I believe the best method may be a technique that has been practiced in the East for centuries. This technique — yoga — not only has remarkable physical benefits, but also emotional and spiritual benefits.

Yoga is — at its simplest — a system for achieving mind-body harmony in which you assume "postures" or "asanas" and practice breathing that enables you to relax and control your body. People who practice yoga regularly report, among other things, that they become more open to problem solving, more creative, less stressed-out by the world around them. Many also report that yoga relieves back pain and strengthens the spine, muscles, and ligaments.

We know for a fact that yoga was in existence at least 2,500 years before the time of Christ, because its practice was recorded in the "Vedas," the oldest books in history. It may have been practiced even before that, however, since even more ancient figures of yogis (practitioners) in meditative poses have been unearthed by scholars and archeologists.

In its purest form, yoga is designed to enable the union of man's individual spirit with the spirit of the universe, or God. This union is achieved by following the "paths" of yoga — Hatha Yoga (which focuses on bodily strength and control), Gnani Yoga (which focuses on knowledge), and Rajah Yoga (which focuses on mastery of the mind).

While yoga is religious in its origins, it need not be practiced like a religion. Millions of people around the world — men and women of all faiths — practice yoga, especially Hatha Yoga, purely for its physical benefits. Viewed as a form of exercise, it is ideal. Yoga can be practiced by anybody. It requires no equipment other than suitable (i.e., comfortable, stretchable) clothing, and it can be practiced at home or in your office — anyplace where there's enough room for you to move without bumping into walls.

The "Sun Salutation"

If I had the ability to somehow "force" you to take just one action to protect yourself from back pain, I'd command you, starting today, to regularly practice yoga — and particularly to practice a single yoga exercise known as the "Sun Salutation."

I myself do this exercise every day and I recommend that all my patients do the same. As far as I'm concerned, this is the single best thing you can do for your back. In addition, it's a great way to deal with stress, to relax, and to achieve mind-body harmony. And it's a great way to warm up before you exercise.

The best time to do the "Sun Salutation" is in the morning or early evening. Start with two sets and work up to six to 10 sets without becoming fatigued or breathing heavily.

Do the 12 positions of the exercise in one continuous, flowing motion, holding each position for five seconds. Your breathing should also be continuous and fluid, connecting the 12 movements — except for one brief pause in breathing when you transition between position 6 and position 7. Inhale (expanding your chest) as you extend your spine, and exhale (contracting your abdomen) as you bend and flex your spine. If you finish the inhale or exhale before you are finished holding a position for five seconds, hold your breath until you start to move into the next position. Be sure to breathe in and out through your nose.

1.   Start in the *Salutation Position*, looking straight ahead and standing straight and tall, with your feet shoulder width apart and your palms together in front of your chest.

[1]:

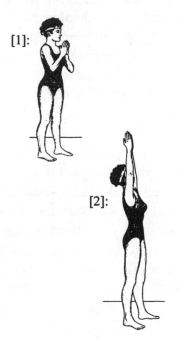

2.   Inhale as you slowly raise your arms up and slightly back in a wide circle, extending your spine and looking up at your hands in the *Raised Arm Position*. Hold for five seconds.

[2]:

3.   Exhale as you bend forward as far as you can into the *Hand to Foot Position* — knees, elbows and shoulders relaxed, and hands flat on the floor or at your ankles (depending on your degree of flexibility). Hold for five seconds.

[3]:

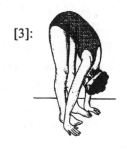

4.   Inhale as you slowly lunge forward with your right leg, lifting your head and spine as you bend your right knee between your arms and extend your left leg back with the left knee touching the floor in the *Equestrian Position*. Hold for five seconds.

[4]:

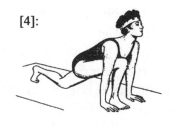

5. Exhale and bring your left leg forward to meet your right leg as you lift your hips and buttocks into the *Mountain Position*, releasing your spine as you press down with your hands, stretch your heels to the floor (feeling the stretch in the backs of your legs), and relax your head and neck. Hold for five seconds.

[5]: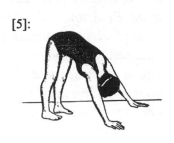

[6]: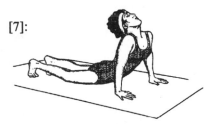

6. Without breathing, bend your knees and elbows and slowly slide your body down, touching your toes, knees, chest hands and chin to the floor in the *Eight Limbs Position*. Hold briefly.

[7]: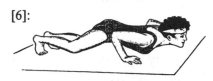

7. Inhale as you lift your head and chest, pressing down with your hands as you arch your back and bring your shoulders down into the *Cobra Position*. Hold for five seconds.

8. Exhale as you repeat the *Mountain Position*, raising your buttocks and hips, and releasing your spine as you press down with your hands. Stretch your heels to the floor (feeling the stretch in the backs of your legs), and relax your head and neck. Hold for five seconds.

[8]: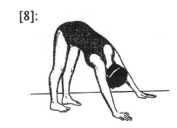

9. Inhale as you repeat the *Equestrian Position*, this time lifting your head and spine as you bring your left leg forward to bend it between your arms, and extending your right leg back with the right knee touching the floor. Hold for five seconds.

[9]: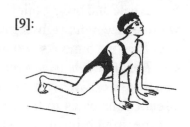

10. Exhale as you repeat the *Hand to Foot Position*, bringing your right leg forward to meet your left leg as you lift your body up and lengthen your spine, keeping your knees, elbows, and shoulders relaxed, and keeping your hands flat on the floor or at your ankles. Hold for five seconds.

[10]: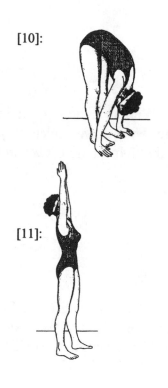

11. Inhale as you repeat the *Raised Arm Position*, lifting your arms straight up and slightly back as you extend your spine and look up at your hands. Hold for five seconds.

[11]:

12. Exhale as you return to the *Salutation Position*, looking straight ahead as you lower your arms and bring your palms together in front of your chest. Hold for five seconds. If you are going to continue with another set, breathe normally in this position for five more seconds before moving into position 2.

[12]: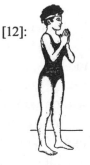

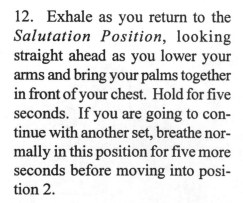

When you have finished your last set, lie flat on your back for two minutes, arms at your sides and palms up, breathing normally.

This routine stimulates all 107 "marma points" of the body (extremely sensitive pressure points used in Indian massage techniques). I call it my "instant feel-good" routine. I know it works for others the same way as it works for me because I've had patients with 20-year histories of back problems who have reported that regular use of the "Sun Salutation" exercise provided complete backache relief.

Additional yoga postures that can help your back

There are other yoga routines you can do that will help your back. These postures, or "asanas," act as a form of mild traction, gently stretching and strengthening the spinal muscles, toning the abdominal organs and stimulating pressure points (marma points) all along the spine. Assume these postures for just a minute or two in the beginning. Then gradually increase the amount of time you devote to each one until you reach the level that gives you the maximum benefit.

[a]:

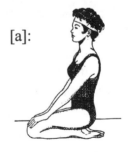

• *The Diamond.* Kneel on a thick carpet or blanket with your knees close together. Sit back on your heels with your hands on your knees, and your back and neck erect. Sit straight so that an imaginary line passing through your ear, shoulder, elbow, and hip would be straight [a]. Inhale as you slowly lift yourself up off your heels, aligning your body straight above your knees [b]. Exhale as you return to the starting posture.

This posture can be used to prepare your body for other postures. It strengthens your back and your pelvic area.

[b]:

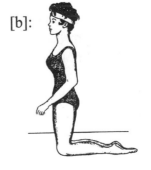

[a]: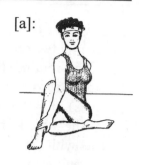

• *The Twist.* Sit on the floor with your right leg bent toward your left hip. Bring your left foot across your right leg, placing it on the floor outside it. Bend your left arm across your lower back with the palm of the left hand facing outwards. Straighten your right arm and bring it across your body, grasping your left ankle from outside your left knee as you twist your body to the left [a]. Exhale. Turn your head and look over your right shoulder. Hold for a few seconds and then twist to look over your left shoulder [b]. (Your shoulders should be at right angles to your body.) Come back to the starting position and repeat on other side.

[b]: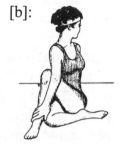

This is a great posture to alleviate lower back pain.

The regular practice of the "Sun Salutation," coupled with the other exercises I talked about in this chapter, gives you a complete "prescription" that you can use to cure your backache quickly, without the use of drugs (in all but the most serious cases) — and then avoid that kind of pain for the rest of your life!

Keep in mind that it can take you anywhere from six months to a year or more to make your back care habitual. The important thing is to continue on with my seven-step program — at your own pace.

In the next chapter, I'll talk about the importance of nutrition and diet, and teach you how to eat right for longevity.

Actions to Take

• Strengthen your back with stretching exercises, as well as weight training. Exercise every day if you already have a back problem — three times a week for prevention. If you have a history of back problems, be sure to include squats and stiff-legged deadlifts in your regimen, and avoid barbell biceps curls, leg curls, and extensions.

• Practice the "Sun Salutation" daily, and experiment with additional yoga postures.

Chapter Eleven

Step 7:
The Substance of Being

Nowhere in the world has nutrition been more carefully analyzed than in the United States. Yet Americans are notorious for poor eating habits — and it seems to be getting worse. We are one of the world's most overweight nations. We have high incidences of heart disease and cancer because we do not view food for its health-associated values. More than 40 percent of Americans take vitamins and nutritional aids, thinking that this lets them off the hook as far as good nutrition is concerned. We have managed to ignore or lose sight of the simple dietary practices that people in much of the rest of the world still follow — good food in moderation.

The wisdom of the East

The Japanese reject our four food groups and choose foods for their yin/yang qualities. Yang foods are from hot and dry environments, so they contain more water, have a strong aroma, and tend to be spicy. Yin foods are from cold and wet climates, so they are dry, hard, sour, and salty. Yang foods are used to bring yin people (those with high mental activity) into balance, and yin foods are used to bring yang people (those who are physically active) into balance.

Ayurvedic practitioners believe that food is the most important means to health. They divide food into six tastes: sweet, sour, salty, astringent, pungent, and bitter. Like the Japanese, Ayurvedic practitioners use food to balance the physiology of the human mind-body. Foods that are sweet, sour, and salty are used to pacify the mentally active "vata" types. Sweet, bitter, and astringent foods are used to calm the fiery "pitta" types. And, finally, the pungent, astringent, and bitter foods are used to activate the somewhat lethargic "kapha" types.

An understanding of the medicinal value of food

Outside of America, food is almost always understood for its medicinal value. Ginger is used in India and China as a digestive aid, and also to relieve nausea, indigestion, heart burn, and the vertigo of motion sickness. Garlic controls infections, colds, flu, hypertension, and cancer. Fenugreek (a leguminous herb with aromatic seeds full of calcium and other minerals) is used in Chinese tea as an aphrodisiac and as a breast cancer preventive.

I could go on for pages and pages with more examples of the way food is used in other cultures to create health rather than to cause disease. In fact, I recently edited *Natural Health Secrets From Around the World*, a 425-page book that offers over 1,200 natural remedies for over 100 common ailments.

If we as a nation are going to reduce our obesity and our high incidence of diseases, we must learn that moderation and balance are the keys to healthy nutrition.

The rules keep changing

Let me say at the outset that there is a problem with teaching nutrition. That's because what we know about the body's requirements is constantly being amended as we acquire more sophisticated data about vitamins, trace minerals, saturated and unsaturated fats, protein, and carbohydrates. Consider, for example, the change in the medical opinion of eggs and red meat in just the last decade or so, and the very recent debate about the ability of beta-carotene to prevent cancer.

I'm sure you remember the time when a "healthy" breakfast consisted of fried eggs, bacon, toast, and juice. Generations of Americans grew up believing that eating a breakfast like this was the right way — the only way — to start their day. Now, of course, we know that bacon and eggs yolks are too high in cholesterol, and that egg consumption should be limited to no more than two or three yolks per week.

And you were probably taught as a youngster that the best dinner starred a thick hunk of steak, and that you should stay away from potatoes because they were considered to be starchy and, hence, "fattening."

Now we know that red meat (and even farm-bred chicken) is loaded with fat from the feed that's given to the animals destined for our dinner plates. We know that potatoes are not fattening, but that the butter and sour cream we use to dress them up are. And that the fat in steak and sour cream and butter is one of the major causes of heart disease, cancer, high blood pressure, and the other ravages of obesity.

What I'll present to you in this chapter is the latest nutritional information I have combined with knowledge derived from my medical studies and from my dealings with my patients. I'll teach you the best way to get the nutrients you need for healthy, zestful living, and how to get and maintain a body that's not carrying around 30 or 50 or 100 pounds of unwanted fatty tissue.

The specific goals of my nutritional program

The primary goals of my nutritional program are health, vitality, longevity, and disease prevention. You'll achieve these goals by following a sensible, rational diet that is low in animal and vegetable fats and high in fiber, complex carbohydrates, and natural antioxidants. This diet will also enable you to lose weight (if you need to), to maintain the right amount of fat and the right amount of muscle, and to keep your weight at the ideal level.

It's that simple.

Why fad diets don't work

A quick word here about fad diets (and that's any diet that has a name, like the "Pound-Buster Diet" or the "Hot Fudge Diet"). Fad diets don't work! Though many of the fad diets you read about or see advertised on television may work in the short run, they don't work long term. They don't achieve the "cure" to obesity — permanent non-obesity.

Fad diets — on which Americans spend billions of dollars every year, seduced by the promise that they'll lose huge amounts of weight in 10 days or two weeks — are not truly diets. They're programs of planned starvation. They strip weight from fat reserves, and also from the muscles by causing a breakdown of proteins in the body (what nutritionists call "negative nitrogen balance"). When the diet is discontinued, the weight almost always comes back. But it returns as fat instead of muscle.

Let's assume you weigh 200 pounds and have 30 percent body fat. That means 60 pounds of your total weight is comprised of fat. If you go on a crash diet and lose 20 pounds, not all of the weight you lose will be from that reservoir of fat. At least part of your weight loss — probably one-third, or 6.6 pounds — will come from muscle.

If, like most dieters, you don't follow up that quick weight loss with a sensible diet, you'll quickly gain back the 20 pounds you lost. But — and this is an important "but" — you will regain it as fat, pushing your total body fat to 33.3 percent, or 66.6 pounds.

There's only one way to safely lose weight

There is only one way to safely take off weight and keep it off while providing your body with all the elements it needs for good health — follow a program of proper nutrition coupled with exercise. That means that you have to eat the proper foods in the proper amounts to give you the vitamins and minerals and nutrient enzymes you need to live in good health, and you need to exercise to utilize your excess body fat as energy. This plan is the keystone that holds my entire seven-step program together.

The dangers of a poor diet

Consider this: Heart disease, cancer, and stroke are the top three killers in the U.S. They account for about 75 percent of the approximately 2 million deaths reported each year. These diseases have been linked, without any doubt, to improper diet. They have been linked to high levels of fat and to a lack of the antioxidants and phytochemicals necessary to ward off changes in the cells that begin the cancer process.

And this: A plethora of other diseases and health problems including obesity, nutritional-variety anemia, gastrointestinal diseases, osteoporosis, and even tooth decay, have been linked to poor dietary habits.

Eat the right foods, and you load yourself not just with the "fuel" you need to break-dance at age 90, but with healthy, disease-preventing antioxidants. Eat the wrong foods and you turn your belly into a sagging mass of pie dough, and your arteries into sludge-filled sewer pipes narrowed to uselessness by free radical damage.

Eat a diet low in animal and vegetable fats and high in fiber, and you "bullet-proof" your body against free radical damage and the illnesses caused by poor dietary choices. Eat a diet high in animal and vegetable fats, and you expose yourself to what one physician-researcher called "a free radical mess."

Eat the right foods in the right amounts, and watch fat melt and turn into lean, trim muscle with exercise. Stuff yourself indiscriminately at each and every meal, and increase your risk of disease and death.

Eat the right foods and extend your life. Put the brakes on aging and force it into full retreat. Eat the wrong foods, and watch your body age and decay before your eyes.

Just how fat is too fat?

I do not always agree with the medical establishment; however, I do agree with a pronouncement made by C. Everett Koop, former Surgeon General of the United States, when he pointed his official finger at obesity caused by poor eating habits and said that it is the number one health problem in the country.

But defining "obesity" is not always easy. It is complicated by our individual perceptions and by the fact that we tend to accept the idea that gaining weight is simply a natural (and unavoidable) part of the aging process.

We are, as a society, so used to people being overweight that we often confuse fat with "normal" and healthy. Dr. George Sheehan, an advocate of running for good health, once said, "If my friends tell me I look good, I know I am too heavy and cannot race or perform as well athletically. If they ask me if I have been sick and say that I look too thin, I know I am at my ideal weight and will be capable of peak performances."

Your ideal weight

There are, of course, charts you can use to pinpoint the supposedly ideal weight for your age, sex, and build or frame size. These are typically promulgated by insurance companies, and are based on statistical averages. However, there are several problems with these charts.

In the first place, these charts figure in data on individuals who don't exercise (the majority of Americans), pushing the averages up. Also, the charts reflect changes in the general population over the last several decades. So, they have gradually allowed higher weights as men and women in our society have, on average, grown heavier. And finally, these charts overemphasize the importance of frame size — whether you're "large boned," "average," or "small-boned" — in determining ideal weight. Your bones and my bones are all the same weight (if we're approximately the same height) when all our other tissues are removed — so the idea of "big bones" and "small bones" is bunk.

In other words, these charts are truly worthwhile only if you want to know the right weight for an overweight, sedentary individual of your age, height, and sex.

Use my formula

A better way to determine your ideal weight is to multiply your height in inches by two. Then add 10 if you are a male, and subtract 10 if you are a female. In other words, a 6-foot male would have an ideal weight of 154 pounds (72 inches x 2, plus 10) and a 5'8" woman would have an ideal weight of 124 pounds (68 inches x 2, minus 10).

I can hear you moaning, saying, "This is ridiculous! I haven't been that weight since I was 18, 19, or 20 years old."

In reality, though, that is the age at which most people achieve their ideal body weight — a weight comprised mainly of lean body mass and little fat. Unfortunately, we have come to accept obesity in mature adults as the norm. We think that a 6-foot male "should" weigh 185 pounds, and that a 5'8" female "looks good" at 145 or 150 pounds. That's just not true. Your ideal weight is the weight you derive using my formula — even if your friends think you're too thin at that weight.

My formula indicates the weight at which you'll be able to perform physically at your very best. It's the weight at which your body fat will be about 10% to 12% of your total weight if you're a male, and about 14% to 16% if you're a female. These are the ideal percentages.

My formula has been adjusted to take into account the fact that fatty tissue weighs more than muscle tissue. As a result, if you use this formula (which I've tested on scores of my patients over the years) and discover that you're at or near your ideal weight — and if you are moderately active — you will also know that this is the weight at which your percentage of body fat is approximately correct.

If, on the other hand, your weight is much higher than your ideal weight — and you can pinch an inch of flesh or more at the back of your arm, about halfway between your shoulder and elbow when your arm is hanging down and loose — chances are your percentage of body fat is higher than it should be.

Body fat is more important than total weight

Because your total weight is less important than your percentage of body fat, my formula will not work for you if you're an athlete who exercises to "bulk up" or add masses of muscle. If, for example, you're a 6'2", 300-pound weight lifter, you would be 142 pounds overweight, according to my formula. Yet your body, while undeniably large, would probably be almost solid muscle. So I certainly would think twice before I called you fat!

The percentage of your total body weight that derives from fat is, indeed, a much more important number for you to know than your total weight. That's the number that tells you whether you're fit or fat.

• For the average man, the normal percentage of body fat is 16% to 18% — for a woman, it's 20% to 22%.

• A man in moderately good shape will have a body-fat percentage in the 12% to 14% range — a woman in moderately good shape will have 15% to 17% body fat.

• A male athlete will have body fat in the 8% to 10% range — a female athlete will have 10% to 12% body fat.

While you can "guesstimate" whether you're at or above these levels, I strongly recommend that you have your body-fat percentage scientifically measured as you begin your program of exercise and diet. That way, you'll have a more exact picture of your true physical condition. And if you have your body-fat percentage measured periodically, you'll have a way to measure your ongoing progress.

Measuring body fat scientifically

If you do decide to have your body-fat percentage measured, it will probably be done with one of these widely used methods, though there are many others:

- *Underwater weighing.* This is the benchmark test, used by athletes for decades.
- *Skin-fold testing, using calipers.* This is the simplest, most common technique.
- *Impedance and fiber-optics tests.* These measure total body water, and calculate body fat using complex computerized formulas.

All of these methods have advantages and disadvantages. Underwater weighing, for example, while very accurate, requires a "dunk tank," and special scales — and can be a problem for people who are uncomfortable when totally underwater. The impedance technique can be troublesome for some men and women because they have to limit their fluid intake prior to testing — and they need to make sure that subsequent tests are all performed at the same time of day to guarantee accuracy. And the accuracy of the skin-fold caliper test depends a great deal on the experience of the tester as well as on the technique used (i.e., three folds, seven folds, etc.).

Furthermore, a study I conducted in 1984 showed that all the major techniques provide no more than an accurate "estimate" of the percentage of your body weight that is fat.

Most nutritionists use either skin-fold caliper or bio-electric impedance tests, despite their drawbacks, because they are simpler to perform than the underwater test — and because test conditions are reproducible. This means that tests can be conducted periodically under exactly the same conditions, and progress can be charted. My personal preference is for the skin-fold caliper test which can be performed on you by your spouse or partner, with a little instruction by any health-care professional, nutritionist, or health club trainer.

You don't have to know your exact body-fat percentage to live a long and healthy life — but you do have to eat right if you plan to stay healthy and active past your 100th birthday.

Lose weight, sensibly

Even if you're out-of-shape, even if you've put on extra pounds, even if your percentage of body fat is excessive and you're suffering from midriff bulge and sagging jowls — you won't have to suffer through a quick weight loss diet prior to starting your program of sensible eating. Unless you are truly obese. Because, if that's the case, your obesity presents an immediate health hazard, and you need to drop 25 or 30 pounds — maybe even more — quickly.

Actually, I think that it's a good idea for any man or woman whose body-fat percentage is 30 percent or more, or who is 30 pounds or more overweight according to my formula to consult with a nutrition counselor for a sensible weight-reduction program.

But remember, this is simply a first step you need to take — for health reasons — before you embark on a nutritional program that will enable you to keep those pounds off forever.

Calories count

Some of the obesity that's endemic in America has as its cause the simple fact that we, as a people, eat too much of the wrong foods. We take in too many calories from fat and simple sugars, and too few from carbohydrates. (A calorie is a measurement of the amount of heat or energy produced by a given amount of any food. This heat or energy is produced by the fat, carbohydrates, and protein found in the food.)

To determine just how many calories you should be taking in each day, start by multiplying your ideal weight (see page 158) by 10 or 11 if you are a man, and by nine or 10 if you are a woman. Then find the sum of that number plus 50 percent.

For example, a man who is 5'10" should weigh 150 pounds, according to my formula. Multiply 150 by 11 to get the number 1,650. The sum of 1,650 plus 50% percent of this number (825) indicates what this man's caloric intake should be to provide him with all the calories he needs for activity and for basal metabolism (calories burned while at rest or asleep): 1,650 + 825 = 2,475. This hypothetical man, then, could consume 2,475 calories per day and maintain his ideal weight.

A 5'2" woman following the same procedure would have an ideal weight of 118 pounds, an ideal basal caloric intake of 1,180 calories (118 x 10) and an ideal total caloric intake of 1,770 calories (1,180 + 590 = 1,770).

The importance of metabolism

Some people take in, in a normal day, more calories than they need. They can lose some weight simply by eating less — no more than their ideal caloric intake.

On the other hand, once body fat exceeds 25 percent in a male and 30 percent in a female, the important factor shifts from how many calories you take in to how your body's metabolism manages the calories you do consume. That is why some people can consume fewer calories than they need — and they're still overweight.

One of the most significant advances made in the study of nutrition in the last decade is understanding that your body adjusts to your caloric intake by either slowing down or speeding up your metabolic rate (the rate at which calories are burned). This explains why a dieter can stay fat while eating only 1,000 calories a day, or even less — the body adjusts to the reduced intake of calories by burning fewer calories.

Shift the source of your calories

More than 90 percent of the men and women who come to me for weight loss consume too few calories, not too many. In fact, I rarely (very rarely) have patients who count calories, because weight and health depend primarily on a balance between nutrition and exercise.

If you were in my office for weight loss and nutrition counseling, the first thing I'd tell you to do is to balance your diet. Then, one step at a time, I'd get you to lower the percentage of calories you get from animal fat, and then to lower the total percentage of your fat calories to the 10% to 15% range. My goal — your goal — must be to get 15% to 20% of your calories from protein, 60% to 70% from complex carbohydrates, and 15% to 20% of your calories (or even less) from fat. By getting less of your calories from fat, you will automatically lose weight without eating less because fat produces about 9 calories per gram of weight — carbohydrates and proteins produce only about 4 calories per gram of weight.

You can't do it without exercise

If your diet is balanced, and you are still overweight, the answer lies not in counting calories, but in speeding up your metabolism and decreasing body fat by becoming more active physically. All too often, I see men and women who want to lose weight before they exercise. It doesn't work. You have to mix proper nutrition and exercise. And I have yet to find a patient, man or woman, who has not been able to perform some kind of safe, health-enhancing physical activity.

Replace body fat with muscle

Your body fat, as you grow older, tends to be deposited like extra baggage. Men, for example, have a tendency to get flabby bellies. Women watch their hips and buttocks grow ever larger. And both men and women suffer from drooping breasts and jowls. Proper nutrition, coupled with aerobic and resistance exercises, can eliminate some of this fat and increase muscle mass.

In some cases you can get rid of sagging flesh and look and feel better without actually changing your body's weight. That is because exercise and a balanced diet, together, decrease your body-fat percentage. If, for example, you weigh 150 pounds and have 25 percent body fat, you're carrying around 37.5 pounds of fat. If you stay at 150 pounds, but reduce your body fat level to just 18 percent, you'll replace more than 10 pounds with muscle mass. You can't help but look better — and feel better about yourself in the process.

Lose weight while you gain strength

The reality of the situation, however, is that most of us need — and want — to lose weight. When I was 225 pounds and out-of-shape, I needed to do more than just tighten my belly and my jowls. I lost the weight, and I feel better and look better today than I did years ago.

If you want to lose the extra pounds you've gained over the years — while you firm and strengthen your body — combine a program of balanced nutrition with exercise. Research has proven that by doing this, you can lose from one-half pound per week to three pounds per week — or between 26 and 156 pounds in just 12 months.

Balance your diet

The typical American diet contains about 40 percent fat, often as much as 35 percent protein (thanks to our penchant for devouring red meat), and only 25 percent carbohydrates. If you are — or have been — making diet choices based largely on convenience and on outdated information, you're short-changing yourself when it comes to carbohydrates, your major source of energy. And if you're not getting enough of your calories from carbohydrates, your body is "stealing" protein from your food intake or from your tissues and converting that protein into energy rather than using it for tissue building and maintenance.

It is easier than you think to provide yourself with the balanced diet you need if you want to stay healthy and live to be 100 or 120 years old. You don't have to give up good eating in order to enjoy healthy eating. In fact, I believe (and preach) that it's possible to both eat to live and live to eat.

• *Complex carbohydrates should account for 60% to 70% of your daily nutritional intake.*

Forget everything you used to know about carbohydrates. They are not fattening — though carbohydrates from cakes and cookies can be unhealthy since they're loaded with sugar. Good sources include fresh fruits and vegetables, legumes (like beans and lentils), whole-grain breads and cereals, and starches (like potatoes, rice, and pasta).

• *Protein should account for 15% to 20% of your daily intake.* Good sources of protein include legumes (also a good source of carbohydrates), fish, poultry, lean red meats, and low-fat dairy products.

• *Fats should account for from 15% to 20% of your daily intake.* Sources of fats include monounsaturated fats (from olive, canola, and peanut oils, avocados, and some nuts), polyunsaturated fats (from corn, safflower, and sunflower oils, margarine, mayonnaise, and most nuts), and saturated fat (mostly derived from animal sources).

Eat moderately and sensibly

You probably need to cut way down on your intake of fatty red meats and high-fat dairy products. And you probably need to lay off the margarine and scrambled eggs, and start eating lots more fresh vegetables and fruits. You need to develop sound dietary habits, and to make sure you have the high-fiber, low-fat foods you need to prevent free radical damage. Here's what I recommend:

- Eat at least three meals a day.
- Eat breakfast every morning.
- Don't eat red meat more than three times weekly.
- Don't eat more than three egg yolks weekly. If you eat more than three eggs, discard the yolks of all but three. If you use eggs in baking or cooking, you can discard two or three yolks without hurting your recipe.
- Drink eight to 10 glasses of water every day.
- Eat three to five whole fruits each day.
- Eat three to four servings of different vegetables each day. (Salad does not count — cooked vegetables are preferred.)
- Eat three slices of whole grain bread (bread in which whole grain flour is listed as the first ingredient) each day.
- Have at least one serving each day of rice, potatoes, or pasta, but preferably more than one. (No butter, margarine, or sour cream.)
- If you are trying to lose weight, limit your meat, fish, or chicken portions to 3 to 4 ounces (not the 6 to 8 ounces you are usually served in a restaurant). If weight loss is not your goal, do not limit portion sizes.
- Limit your caffeine intake to three servings a day. This includes coffee, tea, diet cola, etc.
- Limit coffee, tea, diet soda and other liquids containing artificial sweeteners to no more than three daily — or reduce your total intake of artificial sweeteners to three packets daily. (There is an apparent inhibitory factor in weight loss associated with artificial sweeteners that has, as yet, not been identified.)
- Do not eat cheese more than three times a week — and choose cheeses made from skim milk, like feta, farmer's cheese, or mozzarella.
- Use beans, rice, grains, nuts (other than peanuts), and seeds as a source of protein instead of animal protein. These vegetables also provide minerals and vitamins you won't

get from animal protein.

- Veal, pork, skinned chicken, and fish are better sources of protein than red meat. Fresh ocean fish and free-range chicken are best.
- Eat shellfish in moderation since they are slightly higher in fat content than other fish.

By following my plan, you'll obtain the majority of the recommended daily allowances for vitamins and minerals. It will provide you with 25 to 30 grams of fiber, along with as many of the naturally occurring antioxidants as is possible for you to get from food.

Make intelligent choices

You can go as far as you wish in changing your eating habits. You can — and many individuals I know and respect have done just this — become a dietary reactionary, eating little more than nuts and berries, and cutting out all meats and dairy products. Or you can opt to make just a few changes, perhaps by replacing red meat with fish or chicken in your diet just two or three times a week. You can drink alcohol in moderation, or swear off it forever. You can have ice cream for dessert, or fresh fruit. I drink a couple of cups of coffee each day. You may decide to forego caffeine completely. The choices are yours. The important thing is that you make intelligent, informed choices. That you stop blindly putting food and drink in your belly without paying attention to the impact on your health.

Here are some more facts and figures to help you make decisions about changes in your diet.

- You don't have to count calories as long as your diet is balanced with carbohydrates (60% to 70%), fats (15% to 20%), and protein (15% to 20%).
- Exercise at least 30 minutes a day if you're trying to maximize your weight loss, and exercise 30 minutes three times a week for weight maintenance.
- Since 1890, our diets have shifted from being high in complex carbohydrates to high in fat and simple sugars. The typical American gets about 40% to 45% of his calories from fat, and consumes about 150 pounds of sugar annually.

- Preservatives in food cause free radical damage, so stick to organic products.
- Our nation's soil has changed over time. It has been depleted of the nitrogen necessary for balanced trace-mineral intake, and has been contaminated with chemicals. We can no longer depend on food to provide us with all the vitamins we need. Beta-carotene levels in carrots, for example, vary from bunch to bunch, depending upon where the carrots were grown. For this reason, also, I recommend organically grown products.
- Allegedly "low-fat" foods may derive as much as 80% of their calories from fat, because many manufacturers compute the percentage of fat in their products as a percentage of total weight, including water that has no caloric value. In other words, a product that has 100 calories from fat out of a total of 140 calories should have a represented fat content of about 70%. However, if the weight of the fat in the product is just 10 grams out of a total of 100 grams (including calorie-free water), the product is often represented as being "90% fat free."
- Read labels carefully. The new FDA labeling should prevent the food industry from giving us false or misleading information. Serving sizes are now standardized, total calories are on the label along with the amount of calories and grams of macro nutrients (carbohydrates, fats, and protein), and the breakdown of saturated and unsaturated fat is represented.
- Artificially sweetened and non-fat foods are not necessarily nutritionally good foods.
- Exercise increases your energy needs for hours — altering, in a positive way, how food is used by your body.
- Food is burned as energy. The proper ratio of the macro nutrients that you eat is the key to health through nutrition. If you have too much fat in your diet, your body starts to store it.
- While caffeine and other stimulants will give you an immediate jolt of energy, they lack nutritional value. Broccoli (and other fresh vegetables), on the other hand, won't give you an energy "kick," but they will give you

long-term energy because they're loaded with carbohydrates, vitamins, minerals, and the phytochemicals you need for good nutrition and health. Opt for the long-term benefits.

- Alcohol, artificial sweeteners, and caffeine all alter the body's ability to metabolize fat.
- If it grows on a tree, under the ground, or on a bush — and it's fresh — eat it. In other words, fresh fruits and vegetables are your first choice. Frozen fruits and vegetables should be your second choice. And canned or processed produce should be your third choice. Be aware that not all "fresh" produce found in grocery stores is truly fresh. It may be weeks old. If you can, purchase from a "farmer's market" or a roadside stand.
- If you need to sweeten your food, use Suc-a-Nat (granulated sugar cane), raw sugar, or natural honey to reduce your intake of refined sugar and artificial sweeteners.
- Ideally, you should eat three meals a day. But they don't have to be huge meals in the typically American style. I recommend that you follow the lead of other cultures that have maintained good health and sound nutrition. Eat a light breakfast. Then eat your main meal of the day between noon and 2 p.m. Finish with a light evening meal — and don't eat anything after approximately 8 p.m.

Do it your way

Experience teaches me that when you start eating a healthy diet, you'll be so satisfied that you won't have the appetite for unhealthy foods. It also teaches me that once you start to eat properly, you'll realize how great you feel — and you'll want to make even more changes, gradually, over time.

In my own case, for example, I first tried a vegetarian diet for one month — as a joke — way back in 1977. After that month was up, I realized I felt wonderful, and I haven't had a piece of red meat since that day.

By improving your diet and nutrition — in your own way and at your own speed — you will make a positive step toward determining not just how long you'll live, but also how well you'll age.

In Appendix D, you'll find specific menu recommendations designed to give you an ideally balanced diet.

Actions to Take

• Determine your body-fat percentage and your ideal weight as outlined in this chapter. (Measure your body fat periodically to check on your progress.)

• If you are obese, consult with a nutrition counselor and start on a sensible weight-loss program.

• Determine your true caloric intake by keeping a record of your food intake over a week, and determine your ideal caloric intake using the formula in this chapter. Compare the two numbers, and adjust your intake if necessary.

• Balance your diet to get about 60% to 70% of your caloric intake from complex carbohydrates, 15% to 20% from fats, and 15% to 20% from protein.

• Drink 8 to 10 glasses of water, and eat 3 to 5 whole fruits, 3 to 4 servings of cooked vegetables, 3 slices of whole grain bread, and at least one serving of rice, pasta, or potatoes — every day.

• Continue to exercise.

The Rewards
of Enlightenment

There was a time, not too long ago, when most men and women had to face the prospect of growing older with fear. Why? Because growing older meant growing weaker and being debilitated by illness. And it often meant loss of mental acuity — the loss even of the memories that could serve to make old age at least a time for pleasant reflection.

In these pages, however, you have learned that growing older no longer needs to be the terrifying prospect that it once was. Thanks to *Healthy at 100*, there is a new way to look at aging, and, even more important, there is a new way for us all, including physicians, to approach the aging process.

This new perspective is the direct result of melding Eastern medicine (especially the traditional Ayurvedic medicine of India) and Western medicine — for the first time ever. It is the result of a new understanding of the link between mind and body — a link that we have proven by observing the health benefits of stress management and meditation combined with the latest medical breakthroughs in the particular fields of nutrition and exercise.

In this book, I have given you the very latest information. My recommendations are, in a very real sense, the offspring of this marriage between modern Western science and the ancient healing methods of the East. As a result, I have given you what might be considered a "guidebook" to 21st century medicine.

If you follow the recommendations in these pages — if you take my seven steps to a century of great health — I have no doubt that you will be healthier, happier, and more content. You will be more active, and filled with vitality. And, at the same time, you'll add years to your life.

Keep in mind that the marriage between East and West is still young, and that 21st century medicine is still in its infancy. There is still much to be learned by all of us, scientists and laymen alike, about nutrition, exercise, antioxidant therapies — and about the inviolable link between our minds and our bodies.

That means that by reading this book and putting the information you find in these pages into action in your life, you are just beginning what I hope and trust will be your lifelong search for knowledge about how you can live healthier and longer. (Remember, Ayurvedic means "knowledge of life" — *your* life.)

It's up to you. That, ultimately, is what my seven-step program is really about. You must accept the responsibility for your own health throughout your entire life — even well into what used to be considered "old age."

You are just starting what should be the greatest adventure of your life — your journey to healthy longevity! I trust that what you've learned here will set you on the right course and speed you on your way.

The Seven Steps to a Century of Great Health

1 *Perform your own health-risk assessment.* Examine your heredity as well as risk factors such as smoking, drinking, and lack of exercise. Determine what actions you need to take, or avoid, in order to reduce your risk. See Chapter Five for details.

2 *Start using antioxidants.* Take daily doses of vitamins E, C, and A, along with beta-carotene, and specific nutrients and herbs to fight off the effects of free radicals. See Chapter Six for details.

3 *Practice a form of aerobics for a healthy heart.* Exercise three times a week for 30 minutes each time for just three months. Then make this a habit for the rest of your life. See Chapter Seven for details.

4 *Meditate for stress management and mind-body health.* Meditate at least once daily (twice daily, if possible) for 10 to 20 minutes each session. See Chapter Eight for details.

5 *Practice weight training for stronger bones.* Follow the program I recommend, striving for a balance between free weight exercises and resistance machine exercises (in moderation). See Chapter Nine for details.

6 *Stretch and strengthen your back.* Exercise your back regularly, using the recommended stretching and strengthening exercises, along with the Yoga "Sun Salutation" exercise. See Chapter Ten for details.

7 *Eat right for health.* Follow my guidelines for a balanced, nutrition-rich diet that is high in vitamins, antioxidants, and phytochemicals that fight cancer. See Chapter Eleven for details.

Achieving a Smoke-Free Life

If you're a smoker, there's nothing more important, in terms of your health, than "kicking" your tobacco habit. The tobacco companies' denials notwithstanding, smoking is a killer habit. That's a fact, plain and simple.

It is also a fact, however, that freeing yourself of an addiction to tobacco can be one of the most challenging tasks you can set for yourself. When I quit smoking in 1975, it was one of the most difficult experiences of my life. In truth, the hold of tobacco over many people makes quitting without professional intervention impossible — no matter how strong their motivation.

Over the past 20 years or so, I've helped thousands of men and women begin to live smoke-free lives. In that time, I developed a treatment modality that enables individuals to kick the smoking habit with a minimum of either physical or emotional discomfort, for good and always, with an amazingly high success rate. One of the most important things I have learned is that smokers have a strong addiction and they need understanding and empathy.

I am not saying that it is impossible for you to quit smoking on your own — to go "cold turkey." My experience, however, has shown that simply putting your cigarettes aside and counting on will power, by itself, to free you from your addiction is the least effective way to quit smoking. For that reason, I recommend that you follow the program I developed and use every day at my health clinic in Florida. Every one of my patients who wanted to stop smoking has been successful so long as they continued with follow-up treatment after three, six, and 12 months.

The method I'll teach you will — in all likelihood — enable you to give up cigarettes forever. If you're not able to stop the first time, try again. Don't give up. Many men and women "quit" several times, picking up the habit again before putting down cigarettes for good.

My Program — Step-by-Step

1. Make a list of about a half-dozen reasons you want to quit. This is a list you'll keep and carry in your wallet or purse so that you can refer to it any time you're tempted to light up again.

Your list will be, obviously, personal. It could, though, include such reasons as:
- I want to quit because I'm short of breath.
- I want to quit because my smoking hurts my children.
- I want to quit because I'm sick and tired of my breath and hair and clothes smelling like smoke.
- I want to quit because it's important for me to be in control of my own life.
- I want to quit so I can run better.
- I want to quit to save $3.40 a day.

2. At the same time that you make your first list, make another list that details your smoking habits. In other words, write out just how and when you smoke throughout the day.
- Do you have a cigarette before you get out of bed each morning? If so, you're "habituated" to smoking before you rise. To make non-smoking easier, you'll have to

break that ritual — perhaps by getting out of bed as soon as you wake up and brushing your teeth.

- Do you always have a cigarette and coffee on your work breaks? If you do, you'll have to find a new way to relax. Chew gum and go for a walk outside. Or eat fresh fruit.
- Do you smoke when you're under stress on the job — perhaps right before you make each sales call? If you do, you'll have to break that pattern, too. Deep breathing exercises might help.

3. It is important for you to realize that your smoking addiction has two elements — the psychological need that expresses itself, to a great extent, in your habits or rituals, and the physical need for tobacco/nicotine.

See your doctor for help with your physical addiction. Ask him or her for a prescription for one of the nicotine patches which have been introduced in the last several years. These patches look like square bandages and contain nicotine in varying doses that is absorbed through the skin. They have helped literally millions of Americans quit smoking in just the four years or so that they've been on the market. Since they dispense some nicotine to your system, they eliminate many of the physical symptoms of nicotine withdrawal, including nervousness, irritability, headaches, and sleeplessness.

The typical smoker uses these patches for three or four months, decreasing the strength of the patches (in terms of the amount of nicotine released over every 24-hour period), every month, until the dependence on nicotine abates.

4. As you go through withdrawal — even though it will be eased by the use of the patches — you will find meditation to be helpful, particularly during rough periods. Train yourself to relax when you feel an overwhelming need for a cigarette. Breathe deeply and regularly, and imagine something that you find particularly pleasant or comforting. Perhaps you love sailing, and want to imagine the sight of the sunset as seen over the bowsprit of a gently moving sloop. Or perhaps you love the mountains in winter and can relax (and lessen your need for a cigarette) by visualizing your-

self tucked away in a snow-covered mountain hideaway. You can even visualize how clean and clear your lungs will be or how much younger you'll look as a result of kicking your habit.

Here are some specific tips on using this visualization technique to help you stop smoking:

- Visualize in your mind something that makes you feel good.
- Relax. Close your mouth and inhale slowly and as deeply as possible. Remain relaxed.
- Hold your breath for a four count.
- Exhale slowly, emptying your lungs.
- Repeat these steps five times.

Many of my patients report that performing this simple "ritual" when they feel a strong desire to smoke actually relieves the desire.

The same results can be achieved through hypnosis and, in fact, in my practice, I teach patients how to hypnotize themselves to overcome the urges they have (and that you'll have) while going through the withdrawal process. Unfortunately, I can't teach you self-hypnosis in a book. However, you can get some of the benefits of hypnosis by listening to cassette tapes that combine subliminal messages (messages you're not conscious of receiving) with straightforward messages that provide positive reinforcement. Many patients have success by listening to these tapes while falling asleep — especially when they use the tapes in conjunction with nicotine patches, and the meditation-visualization technique I described above. The tapes are available at many health food stores and bookstores.

5. <u>You must exercise when you are trying to quit smoking.</u> Aerobic exercise, particularly walking at a brisk pace or jogging, five to six times a week for 20 to 30 minutes per session, help reduce stress, and make you feel better about yourself and your health as you work toward becoming smoke-free.

6. <u>Some other techniques you can use if you need a little extra help in the beginning</u>:

- Keep your hands busy. Knit or sew, write a letter, take up wood-carving, or work on a jigsaw puzzle or your computer.

- Spend time with non-smokers. If you're trying to quit, stay away from places where smokers congregate.
- If you're going to a place where you know many people will be smoking, plan ahead. Imagine how good you'll look, how good the food will taste, how much better your clothes will smell if you don't smoke. Give your self positive reinforcement.
- Practice the "Four Ds":
  Delay: The urge to smoke will pass, whether you light up or not.
  Deep breathe: It'll help you relax.
  Drink water: It makes the urge to smoke easier to handle.
  Do something: Do anything to get your mind off smoking.

7. If you find it impossible to quit with the help I've given you in these pages, run, don't walk, to get the personal, "hands-on" help of a specialist in treating addictions. There's nothing at all to be ashamed of if you need help when you take this life-saving step. Many people find it necessary to work in partnership with a specialist who has additional ways to make the quitting process as easy as possible.

Healing Yourself Naturally

In my private practice, there's nothing I enjoy more than teaching my patients that they have the power to heal themselves. I see myself as a facilitator and educator whose primary function is to convince patients that real healing comes from within — whether they're facing something as simple as back strain or something as terrifying as cancer.

Many studies have shown that patients who acknowledge that power experience significant physiological changes — from lower blood pressure to greater immune function — that help them heal.

With that in mind, here are some of my best "home remedies" for four of the more common ailments I see among my patients.

HEADACHE
There's an old saying that there's nothing certain in life except death and taxes. Well, add headache to that. According to a recent

study, 93 percent of men and 99 percent of women will have a headache at least once in their lives. For nine out of 10 of them, it will be a tension headache — that dull ache that feels like a vise is slowly being tightened around your head. About 18 million people will suffer from migraine — a throbbing, blinding headache frequently accompanied by nausea and vomiting. And about a million will experience a cluster headache — so excruciatingly painful that some describe it as feeling like a red-hot poker is being driven through the skull. (It has been known to make grown men cry.)

About 50 million Americans see their doctors every year for headaches and spend about half a billion dollars annually for pain medications — some of which is unnecessary, and, in fact, may be doing more harm than good.

If you're constantly popping aspirin or ibuprofen for headache, you're risking kidney and liver damage. You're also building up a tolerance to these analgesics, and, chances are, you're going to ask your doctor for something more powerful — and potentially more dangerous and addicting.

In my practice, I've found that many headaches — even migraines — respond well to simple lifestyle changes and to natural treatments and remedies (everything from avoiding certain foods to self-applied acupressure). But before I make my recommendations for self-treatment, I first rule out an organic cause.

Though less than one percent of headaches have organic causes, you should always consult your doctor before you try to treat yourself. Make sure you aren't suffering from a physical problem (such as a brain tumor) or that your headache isn't the legacy of an earlier trauma (such as a blow to the head), which will require medical treatment.

For severe headaches that don't respond to self-care, I refer my patients to a good headache specialist whose medical arsenal may include everything from antidepressants and analgesics to hypnotherapy and biofeedback. To locate a headache specialist in your area, write or call the National Headache Foundation, 5252 North Western Avenue, Chicago, Illinois 60625; 800-843-2256.

But if you're like most people, you'll be able to banish your headaches — sometimes before they start — without reaching for drugs. Experiment with these proven techniques until you find the ones that work for you:

Keep a headache diary

When you have a headache, write a detailed account of what you're doing, what you're thinking, how you're feeling, how long you slept, what you ate, drank — even the weather. Often, if you can pinpoint the cause of your headaches, you can pinpoint a cure.

For example, some people develop headaches if they have too little or too much sleep. Altering their sleep patterns usually cures their headaches.

People who suffer from weekend headaches are often surprised to learn that they're going through withdrawal from their drug of choice — caffeine. They may sleep later on weekend mornings, delaying that first cup of coffee and incurring the dull headache that's the result of not getting a daily dose of caffeine on time.

Some people have what are called "ice cream headaches" — pain triggered when they eat or drink something cold that strikes a nerve in the roof of the mouth. Others get headaches from bright sun, from prolonged exercise, loud noises, acrid smells, the hot dry winds of summer, or the bright cool air of spring and fall.

Once you find the link to your headache, you will probably be able to do something about it. Below are some of my remedies for a few of these common headaches.

Avoid known headache-trigger foods

Chocolate, aged cheeses, fermented foods such as pickles and hot dogs, foods containing monosodium glutamate (MSG), and wine are the best-known headache triggers — but every year new research adds more foods to the list. Other foods known to cause headaches are wheat, nuts, vinegar, avocados, citrus fruits, milk and milk products, eggs, beef, sugar, yeast, bananas, pork, caffeinated beverages, onions, and broad beans.

But that doesn't mean that you have to eliminate all of these offending foods from your diet. They don't all trigger headaches in everyone. For example, you may find you have no problem eating brie and sipping red wine at a cocktail party, while a freshly baked dinner roll gives you a migraine. Use your headache diary to pinpoint the particular foods that cause your headaches.

Try relaxation techniques

Tension headaches, not surprisingly, respond very well to re-

laxation techniques. At most headache centers, specialists use biofeedback and physical therapy instead of drugs to treat these headaches — which are often chronic.

I consider Transcendental Meditation to be good for whatever
ails you, but you can also use five to 10 minutes of progressive
muscle relaxation several times a day to forestall tension headaches:
Find a comfortable chair or couch and close your eyes. Begin with
your toes. Tense them for two seconds, then release the tension.
Move to your heels, then to your ankles and calves, and continue
on — all the way up to your scalp.

Here's another excellent tension-relieving exercise, often recommended for pain due to stress-induced temporal mandibular jaw
(TMJ) disorder: Sitting comfortably in a chair, drop your head to
your chest, pressing your hand firmly but gently against the back
of your head to really stretch the muscles on the back of your neck.
Then drop your head backwards, pressing your hand firmly but
gently on your forehead to stretch the front neck muscles. Drop
your head to one side, again using a firm but gentle touch to stretch
the muscles on the outer part of your neck. Then do the other side.
Repeat each exercise three times and do them three times a day.

Give up caffeine

Give up caffeine, but be forewarned — if you go cold turkey,
you will most assuredly get a headache. The first three days you
go without caffeine, you will probably have a constant, dull headache that's the result of rebound dilation of blood vessels in your
head. To avoid this, I recommend that you taper off caffeinated
beverages (including tea, soft drinks, and chocolate drinks, in addition to coffee). Gradually decrease the number of cups or glasses
you drink each day until you're caffeine-free.

Try a pair of sunglasses

Buy a pair of sunglasses with a 99 percent ultraviolet filter coating. (You can also have your current sunglasses treated with this
coating.) This will help eliminate light-induced headaches.

Avoid alcohol and cigarettes

Drinking and smoking are common triggers of cluster headaches — so quit!

Exercise

While there is a small group of people who get so-called exertional headaches — from running, coughing, even sex — most headache sufferers benefit from a regular exercise program. Why? No one is really sure, but I'm convinced endorphins play a role. Exercise increases the body's production of these chemicals, which are known to relieve pain and lift mood. Regular exercise also helps you sleep better, which will fight those headaches caused by lack of rest. It's also an excellent technique for reducing tension.

Even people who have exertional headaches can take advantage of the healing power of exercise if they do a five to 10 minute warm-up before exercising, and have a brief cool-down period afterward. Walking is a good cool-down exercise, because it draws blood from the cranial region (increased blood flow there can trigger a migraine) to the lower extremities. If you're susceptible to these kinds of headaches, avoid exercising in the middle of the day on warm days, and don't exercise while you have a headache, since that will simply increase your pain.

Check your medicine cabinet

Some drugs can bring on headaches, including oral contraceptives and some heart medications. If, when compiling your headache diary, you notice a connection between a drug you're taking and headache, bring it to the attention of your doctor. You may need a different dosage — or a different drug.

Use an ice pack

Many headache sufferers find relief by pressing an ice pack to the back of their necks, foreheads, or scalps. Never apply ice directly to the skin, because it can cause frostbite.

Apply heat

·While it sounds contradictory to recommend both ice and heat, the truth is that every headache is different. Some sufferers swear by ice, others by a warm pack or a hot shower. Experiment to determine which is right for you.

Try acupressure

There are several points on the body that, when pressed firmly

but gently, can relieve headache pain. Try pressing these points —
for 30 seconds to two minutes — when a headache strikes:
  • the hollow between the two vertical neck muscles at the
    base of the skull
  • the hollow in the center of the back of the head
  • the indentation between the eyebrows where the bridge of
    your nose meets your forehead
  • both sides of the nose at the points where the bridge meets
    your eyebrows
  • the points at the bottom of your cheekbones that directly
    line up with your pupils

SEXUAL VITALITY

When it comes to sexual vitality, all the news is good. As long
as you are healthy, you can have an active sex life until you're 100
and beyond. And you don't have to eat stewed tiger's penis, as
some Asians do, to rekindle the fire if it occasionally sputters. There
are plenty of potent aphrodisiacs that don't cost $500 an ounce.

Rule out an underlying medical problem

The first thing you should do if you've lost your passion or
your potency is to see your doctor for a physical examination. There
are a number of underlying medical conditions that can affect sexual
desire and functioning, and most can be corrected through simple
measures.

In men, for example, vascular insufficiency can lead to impotence by reducing blood flow to the genitals. So can diabetes. For
women, menopause can bring with it a loss of libido (although
some women report an increase in sex drive) and vaginal dryness
that can make intercourse painful. There are even some commonly
used drugs that can undermine your love life, such as blood pressure medications and antihistamines.

Understand the changes that come with age

Aging also brings with it many changes in sexual functioning
for both men and women, and your doctor will be able to help you
sort out what's normal from what's not.

For example, it's normal for both sexes to take longer to become aroused and reach climax — blood flow to the genitals may

decrease. Men may have trouble having and maintaining an erection. The lower level of testosterone that older men have — yes, men, like women, experience a drop in sex hormone production as they age — may be accompanied by a drop in sexual desire. And women may experience a decrease in tactile sensation.

Despite all this, your sex life may get even better as you age. It did for most of the people who responded to a recent national study of older adults. A full 80 percent of the women and 64 percent of the men said sex felt as good as or better than it did when they were younger.

Ask your doctor about testosterone

Scientists are beginning to think of testosterone as the hormone of love — for both men and women. In both sexes, testosterone production falls off as we age, and may be responsible for the loss of libido some older people report. Ironically, it's now believed that the reason some women experience increased libido during and after menopause is that the loss of estrogen allows what little testosterone they produce to take center stage.

Because the research is so new — and so scanty — few doctors are prescribing testosterone along with estrogen replacement therapy for their female patients unless they have had a complete hysterectomy (removal of uterus and ovaries). That's probably because the ovaries continue to produce male hormones for a time after menopause in about half of all women. But it's worth discussing with your doctor. And make sure you ask about side effects. Some women grow excess hair and get acne, which can often be reversed simply by lowering the dosage.

Men should absolutely consider testosterone injections. I have found that some men need only one or two injections to restore them to full sexual functioning. Once they realize that their potency problems have a hormonal basis, it all comes back — without the need for further injections. What's at work here? I believe it's the amazing power of mind over matter.

Weigh the positives and negatives of estrogen replacement

While estrogen doesn't seem to affect sexual desire in women, it does restore the lubrication and elasticity to the post-menopausal vagina. This eliminates a frequent cause of sexual problems in older women — painful intercourse. Estrogen has a few other pluses going for it, including reducing a woman's risk of heart disease and osteoporosis.

But estrogen poses some potential dangers too, including an increased risk of uterine cancer and possibly breast cancer. For this reason, I recommend trying other, safer methods of restoring sexual functioning before turning to estrogen replacement. These include:

• *Progest Cream.* This is a natural extract of the Mexican yam and is available without a prescription. It's the only form of progesterone, another sex hormone, that is identical to the chemical form of progesterone in your body. It's absorbed through the skin and doesn't have any major side effects. There's at least one study that shows it also increases bone density.

• *Replens.* Used three times a week, this over-the-counter cream can restore lubrication and normal pH to the vagina, and also cut down on yeast infections.

• *Enjoy sex frequently.* There are studies that show that women who have and enjoy sex frequently — even masturbation — keep their vaginas naturally lubricated.

• *DHEA.* The adrenal hormone called dehydroepiandrosterone (DHEA) decreases as men and women age and may contribute to driving your passion underground. Ask your doctor to check your DHEA level. If it's low, your doctor may want you to replace it orally with prescription medication every other day. As a bonus, DHEA will keep your body fat normal, and will reduce many of the signs and symptoms of aging. However, there is also evidence that the DHEA supplement decreases the body's own production of this hormone — so it's not a drug to be taken lightly.

Do-it-yourself tips

Try these recommendations to keep your sex life sizzling:

• Go "semi-vegetarian." I prescribe a three-month pseudo-vegetarian diet to my patients with sexual problems to see whether diet makes a difference for them. I let them eat fresh fish and free-range chicken, but nothing raised on factory farms where there are all sorts of contaminants in the feed (like antibiotics, which I'm convinced can lead to sexual dysfunction).

• Avoid fatty foods. A University of Utah study found that

men who eat fatty meals curb their production of testosterone by as much as 30 percent. It's usually a short jump from eating fat to getting fat — and men who have a lot of body fat also have less testosterone. They also risk developing clogged arteries, including the arteries in the penis, which can lead to impotence.

• Take supplements and eat foods containing vitamin E and zinc, both of which are associated with improved sexual functioning. Vitamin E is contained in vegetable oils, whole-grain foods, wheat germ, nuts, and leafy green vegetables. If you're taking supplements, take 200 to 400 International Units (I.U.s) daily.

You'll find zinc in meat and dairy products, oysters, eggs, and legumes. If you're taking supplements, take 80 milligrams.

• Exercise. Study after study shows that exercise is a turn-on for men and women of all ages. One survey of more than 8,000 women found that 40 percent of those who exercised three times a week for three months — my Rule of 3s — were more easily aroused. 27 percent were more orgasmic, and 31 percent had sex more frequently.

Another study found that middle-aged men who exercised at 75 to 80 percent of capacity three to four days a week for nine months had more sex than those who exercised by walking slowly.

How can exercise be such a potent aphrodisiac? Well, for one thing, it increases testosterone levels in men and increases blood flow to the whole body, including the genitals. It improves your mood, boosts your self-esteem, and gives you good feelings about your body. People who participate in exercise programs report fewer sexual frustrations. And running seems to have an edge over walking. In surveys, runners have more sexual desire, arousal, and orgasms than walkers and people who are sedentary.

• Relax. Sex itself is a great way to relax, but many couples can't take advantage of it because they're tensed to the max. Transcendental Meditation is the best form of relaxation because its effects are cumulative. By practicing TM 20 minutes in the morning and 20 minutes at night, you will eventually train your body and mind to feel relaxed all the time, not just 40 minutes a day. Exercises which combine mind-body relaxation are very effective in releasing the tension that blocks passion. Yoga, t'ai chi, and even karate can put your mind and body in the mood.

• Check your medicine chest. There are quite a few drugs

that are known to affect libido and potency — some of which you may be taking. These include antidepressants (particularly Prozac), blood pressure medications (particularly beta-blockers, alpha-blockers, and diuretics), antihistamines, ulcer medications, and antipsychotics.

In many cases, reducing the dosage of the drug you're taking will be enough. In other cases, you may want to switch to another drug. If you have high blood pressure, for example, you may want to ask your doctor to try a calcium channel blocker, which isn't associated with sexual dysfunction.

• Lighten up on work. One of the most common reasons couples lose that loving feeling is that they're just too tired. If you have to, schedule time for sex. If it's written on your calendar, you can take advantage of one of the best forms of foreplay I know — anticipation.

• Be caring. A warm romantic kiss once or twice a day, a half dozen hugs, or doing something unexpected for your partner will all keep the home fires burning and work on your primary sexual organ — your brain. For women especially, sexual satisfaction is linked to a feeling of closeness in a relationship. It's been proven that the majority of couples suffering from inhibited sexual desire have a relationship problem, rather than a sexual problem.

• Do something different. Variety is the spice of your sex life too. So be creative. How about a nice oil massage after a hard day? (The best oils are those designed for massage, rather than baby oil, which can clog pores.) How about taking a weekend away once a month? And, though it may be cramped, how about trying that old standby of teenagers everywhere — the back seat of your car? One couple I know hired a babysitter and spent a nice romantic evening at their local lovers' lane. If all else fails, just move your bedroom furniture around. Or try some completely different positions.

• Avoid alcohol. Ironically, while alcohol may stimulate your desire, it will definitely impede your performance. It can cause impotence in men and delay orgasm in women.

• Try these natural aphrodisiacs recommended by herb experts: wild yams, licorice, oysters, winter cherry, and molucca bean. They're available from your local supermarket or health food store.

PREMENSTRUAL SYNDROME (PMS)

Although surveys have found that 90 percent of all women experience some kind of bothersome symptom before their periods — anything from cramps to melancholy — no woman has to suffer from this "normal" monthly misery. The causes of PMS remain as mysterious as those of a rare disease. But in recent years, one theory is beginning to emerge — PMS is caused by low levels of a brain chemical called serotonin.

Researchers have been drawn to this theory because serotonin-raising drugs — like the antidepressant medication Prozac — also cure many PMS symptoms in most women who have them. Serotonin is the brain chemical that helps you sleep, regulates your sex hormones, alters your mood, and regulates your appetite (specifically for carbohydrates). So you can see how low levels might make you depressed, angry, and prone to sleepless nights and food binges, all common symptoms of PMS.

Studies have shown that women with PMS do have lower than average serotonin levels. And studies indicating that vitamin B6 and magnesium supplements are helpful in some women with PMS, also point to serotonin. Low magnesium tends to interrupt the action of serotonin in the body, and B6 acts like an enzyme in converting the amino acid tryptophan (which we get in food) into serotonin in the brain.

Eat carbohydrates

Fortunately, serotonin is one of the brain chemicals that has been studied extensively, and we know something very important about it. We know that we can increase serotonin in our bodies by eating carbohydrates. So, I would venture to say that almost any woman who sticks to my basic eating plan is going to see a rapid amelioration of most of her premenstrual symptoms.

Exercise

Exercise is good for everything else — and it's proven to be good for PMS symptoms too. Studies have shown that women who exercise regularly are less likely to have PMS, probably because they're stimulating the body's natural pain- and mood-regulators — the endorphins. (Some research has found that endorphins decrease in premenstrual women.)

Cut out caffeine

Studies have found that women who use caffeine are more likely to have PMS. Cut back gradually to avoid caffeine withdrawal symptoms (like headaches).

Avoid salt

It is particularly important for women who tend to retain water and experience "bloating" to avoid salt.

Eat foods high in magnesium, or take supplements

Studies have shown that magnesium supplements can relieve PMS mood swings. In one study, subjects who experienced relief from some of their nastier symptoms were given 360 milligrams of magnesium three times a day. When I read this study, I realized why one woman I know swears her homemade trail mix is a PMS cure — because magnesium-rich foods include nuts and seeds, whole grains, and legumes. Try trail mix — and make your own like my friend does to avoid the salt and candy you often find in store brands.

Try B6

A number of studies have found B6 to be effective, while others have found it to be of little use. I suspect that it is most effective in combination with a high carbohydrate diet because of the role it plays with dietary tryptophan in serotonin production. However, do not take more than 200 milligrams daily. Too much B6 can cause nerve damage.

Ask your doctor to check your iron level

A recent U.S. Department of Agriculture study found that low levels of iron were associated with mood disturbances and pain in women with severe menstrual symptoms. You may need an iron supplement, especially if you aren't eating much red meat. Surveys have found that many menstruating women are deficient in iron, not only because of their eating habits, but because they lose iron with their menstrual flow.

Add some high carbohydrate snacks to your diet

One of my patients refers to the week before her period as "hungry week." We now suspect that premenstrual bingeing is the body's craving for carbohydrates, which it can convert into serotonin. I'm a proponent of paying attention to body wisdom, as long as what your body wants is truly wise. A doughnut is a high carbohydrate snack, but it's loaded with fat and sugar, which will not do your body — or your symptoms — any good. Sugar may even increase your mood swings. Snack on carbohydrates, but stick to good snacks — whole grain breads, crackers, muffins or cereal, fresh fruit and vegetables, and nuts and dried fruits. At this time of the month, you may even want to alter the way you eat. Instead of eating three substantial meals a day, eat six small meals jam-packed with carbs.

Avoid artificial sweeteners
Artificial sweeteners tend to keep the tryptophan in your diet from entering the brain to produce serotonin — so avoid them.

Try evening primrose oil
A number of studies have found that evening primrose oil (found in health-food stores) can ease breast tenderness.

Take ibuprofen
Ibuprofin is good for headache and cramps — and it has certain properties that also make it effective against lesser-known PMS symptoms (like diarrhea).

Try relaxation techniques
While many PMS symptoms have a physical cause, stress can exacerbate them. Transcendental Meditation, yoga, progressive muscle relaxation, deep breathing, or visualization — done regularly — may help relieve the psychological symptoms that precede your period. Some women also swear by biofeedback.

Expose yourself to full-spectrum light for two hours a day
One study turned up a link between PMS and Seasonal Affective Disorder (SAD), the depression some people get during the winter months when they're exposed to less sunlight. Researchers found that some women with PMS, like those suffering from SAD, have decreased production of a hormone called melatonin, pro-

duced by the tiny pineal gland in reaction to light. When the women got two extra hours of artificial full-spectrum light, which is like sunlight, their psychological symptoms improved. Try it.

HAIR LOSS

Thinning hair or impending baldness is not life-threatening, but it's a big problem for many people. That's why drug companies are scrambling to find a cream, lotion, or pill that can restore sparse hair to the thick mane of youth.

For most people (men far more often than women), hair loss is something that's been written into their genes as surely as blue eyes or a dimpled chin. If you're going to lose your hair because of genetics, it's most likely to start between the ages of 18 and 35. The earlier it starts, the faster hair falls out. By the time you reach your mid-40s, you're probably just about done losing what you're going to lose.

But heredity is not the only reason for shedding hair. Medications — common ones like oral contraceptives, anabolic steroids, some cholesterol-lowering drugs, some arthritis medications, beta-blocker blood pressure drugs, and sometimes even commonly prescribed ulcer drugs like Tagamet, Zantac, and Pepcid — can have this unwanted (though temporary) side effect. And hair can fall out as a result of iron deficiency, thyroid disease, a vitamin and mineral deficiency, fad diets, and severe stress (like the death of a loved one, or an ugly divorce). Though, in many of these cases, a simple lifestyle change can turn the problem around.

Care for the hair you still have

Right now, there's no magic potion that can completely restore what you've lost. But there is help for the hair-impaired. There are a number of things you can do to help preserve the hair you have.

- Comb your hair gently when wet, and brush it only when dry.
- Avoid using a hot dryer on your hair. Let it partially air dry first, so you can use your hair dryer for less time.
- Choose hair styles that don't pull on your hair. That means tight pony tails, corn rows, or braids are out if you want to reduce the stress on your hair.
- Consider coloring your hair, but not necessarily to change the color. Hair dyes actually coat the hair strands so that

what you have looks fuller. A permanent can do the same thing. But make sure you go to a professional who knows what he or she is doing and knows the proper precautions to take.

- Shampoo your hair frequently — even every day if it tends to be oily. Greasy hair is heavy and tends to lie down and stick together, making what you have appear thinner. Washing away the oil allows each hair shaft to stand away from the scalp, giving a much fuller appearance.

- Try using Nutriol. This product, available from Nuskin in Provo, Utah, revitalizes the hair shafts and follicles. It won't grow hair if the follicle is already gone, but it may preserve the hair you still have. Nutriol contains proteins, amino acids, vitamin C, biotin, and a few other ingredients. The company recommends that you apply it to your hair and scalp every other day, but I just use it about four times a year as preventive maintenance.

- Add black currant oil to your diet — 500 milligrams twice a day. Andrew Weil, M.D., the author of *Natural Health, Natural Medicine*, says black currant oil is naturally rich in a substance called GLA (gamma-linolenic acid), which is especially helpful for dry, brittle, or thinning hair. But you'll have to be patient. Dr. Weil says that it takes six to eight weeks to see results. After you see improvement, however, you can cut the dose in half. GLA can be used indefinitely.

- Try using sage tea as a rinse. Herbal medicine specialists say this may help hair grow.

- Make sure you are taking an ample supply of vitamins and minerals every day. Healthy hair requires a healthy body. The B vitamins and vitamin E, for example, are important for the health and growth of hair. And the mineral zinc has been shown to stimulate hair growth by enhancing immune function.

Consider minoxidil

It may not be the answer for everyone, but check with your doctor to see if minoxidil (brand name, Rogaine) is right for you.

- Minoxidil is the only drug right now that is approved by the FDA for hair growth. The drug works by blocking the gene which tells hair follicles to shrink, so it's much more effective at stopping hair loss than at growing new hair. In fact, hair experts report that Rogaine stops hair loss in 90 percent of cases. Meanwhile, 70 percent of people get some regrowth, 35 percent show noticeable hair thickening, and 10 percent experience dramatic improvement — all of which takes about 6 months of twice daily applications. The downside is that Rogaine is expensive — about $40 per month to maintain results — and you must use it indefinitely to keep your new hair.

- Ask your dermatologist about minoxidil in combination with retinoic acid (Retin-A). Studies show that the combination of Rogaine and the popular acne medication called Retin-A results in far superior hair growth than minoxidil alone for typical male pattern baldness. And the higher the concentration of Rogaine when mixed with the retinoic acid, the better the outcome.

Promising new products

Scientists are testing many new substances that have the potential to mark the end of involuntary baldness — some say in as little as 5 to 10 years. Here's the latest.

- Cyoctol. This drug, when applied to the scalp, inhibits scalp androgen receptors. Genetic male pattern baldness is dependent on circulating androgens (male hormones), and if those hormones are effectively blocked, then hair loss should be halted or reversed. In one experiment, 82 percent of the men using Cyoctol for a year showed an increase in hair growth, and another 10 percent stayed the same.
- Proscar. This is another anti-androgen, but in pill form. Right now its only approved use is as a treatment for an enlarged prostate. However, Proscar has also shown some effect against male pattern baldness, which is the reason it is now being studied at New York University. Apparently, the excitement surrounding this drug is that it doesn't inhibit all androgens, just the ones that cause baldness.
- Tricomin. This peptide-copper combination was found to grow thick hair on mice. It was discovered by a company called ProCyte in Kirkland, Washington, which, recogniz-

ing its potential, decided to test it on balding men. In one test, 83 percent of those who got the strongest dose grew thicker hair than they had prior to its use — and there were no side effects.

- Hyaluron. This preparation, which consists of hyaluronic acid, glycoproteins, and amino acids, appears to slow the rate of hair loss in the early stages of male pattern baldness. In one French study, hair loss decreased by 59 percent in those using Hyaluron, but decreased by only 16 percent in those using a placebo (drugless substitute). So far, there is no evidence that Hyaluron will grow new hair.

- Spironolactone. This is a common prescription diuretic which may help women, in particular, who have thinning hair due to a sensitivity to certain male hormones that are found in the female body. When taken orally, Spironolactone reduces the activity of these hormones. In one small study of six women, the drug stopped hair loss in four and promoted hair growth in the other two. Spironolactone is now being tested on men — but in a topical formulation that gets rubbed onto their heads. That's because taking it in pill form could alter their male hormones in an unacceptable way.

- Cryotherapy. Researchers in Lisbon, Portugal, tested cryotherapy on a group of men and women with genetic hair loss and determined that moderate cosmetic benefits were seen in 80 percent of the men and 62 percent of the women. The treatments consisted of weekly applications of liquid nitrogen sprayed onto the head for 60 to 90 seconds until the scalp turned red. The researchers think cryotherapy may work because it increases circulation and causes direct stimulation of hair follicle cells. It's also possible that it causes a metabolic change that interferes with the action of androgens on the hair follicles.

Revolutionary Research

In Chapter Eleven, I mentioned that nutrition is a tricky subject because the rules keep changing as we get more sophisticated data from researchers working in the field. One researcher who I believe just may be changing the course of nutrition in America is Barry Sears, Ph.D., a former research scientist at the Boston University School of Medicine and the Massachusetts Institute of Technology. Dr. Sears is a leading expert in intravenous drug delivery technology. His research is based upon viewing nutrition from the perspective of drug delivery technology and hormonal response.

Dr. Sears claims that most of our emphasis on nutrition has been focused on micronutrients, vitamins, and minerals, but that the most important dietary factor is the hormonal response in our bodies that is created by the macronutrient composition of our food. His research indicates that it is the ratio of macronutrients in a meal — in particular the ratio of proteins to carbohydrates, their rates of entry into the bloodstream, and the resulting hormonal responses they generate — that is the most important ingredient in a healthy, balanced diet.

The biological zone theory

The macronutrient balance in Dr. Sears' program calls for 40 percent of calories from low-glycemic carbohydrates (meaning carbohydrates that do not raise blood sugar), 30 percent of calories from protein, and 30 percent of calories from fat (with minimal saturated fat content). According to Dr. Sears, the ratio of protein to carbohydrate at every meal should be between 0.6 to 1.0, with the ideal being 0.75. It is within these protein-to-carbohydrate ratios that powerful hormonal responses are generated that regulate blood sugar levels, allow access to stored body fat for energy, and, most importantly, produce "good" eicosanoids that provide the ultimate hormonal protection against disease.

A genuine breakthrough

This is probably the first time you've ever heard of "eicosanoids," but I predict that you'll be hearing a lot more about them in the future. If Dr. Sears' theory proves out, we're talking about a genuine breakthrough in the field of preventive medicine.

In technical terms, eicosanoids represent a broad spectrum of hormone-like substances including prostaglandins, thromboxanes, leukotrienes, lipoxins, and a variety of fatty acids. What you need to know about them now is that in 1982, the Nobel Prize in Medicine was awarded for work with eicosanoids in the field of human health — and that good eicosanoids have been shown to fight virus infections, inhibit tumor growth in cancer patients, and control diabetes and heart disease. On the other hand, "bad" eicosanoids promote the development of these same disease states.

The biological zone theory especially appeals to me because it is being studied in humans rather than in animals — and the results are very promising. It also appeals to me because it explains why some people who eat a high starch diet (pasta, potatoes, bread, and rice) cannot seem to lose weight, and often have hypoglycemic attacks. With Dr. Sears' eicosanoid-favorable diet, cholesterol falls, blood sugar is maintained, body fat approaches normal, sports performance is improved, and the level of certain cancer fighting hormones rises in the bloodstream.

The eicosanoid-favorable diet

The eicosanoid-favorable diet is very easy to follow for both vegetarians and meat-eaters alike. All you need to do is:

1. Reduce the intake of carbohydrates that have high glycemic indexes, such as pasta, bread, potatoes, rice, and carrots, in favor of low-glycemic carbohydrates (fruits and fiber-rich vegetables) that do not affect the blood sugar as readily.
2. Consume adequate protein to maintain your lean body mass. This means consuming no more protein than your body requires, but never consuming any less (which would represent protein malnutrition).
3. Include enough fat in your diet to allow for the production of good eicosanoids, which are derived from Omega-6 fatty acids, and include additional amounts of Omega-3 fatty acids, which help prevent the overproduction of bad eicosanoids.

Look to the future

Though the biological zone theory, at first glance, appears to be in conflict with my current nutritional recommendations, in many ways both programs have broad areas of similarity. Both programs emphasize fruits and fiber-rich vegetables as carbohydrate sources. Both programs emphasize the need to keep *total* fat consumption low. Both programs emphasize the need for adequate protein in the diet. The primary difference in the programs is that the eicosanoid-favorable diet reduces the total amount of carbohydrates (primarily high-glycemic ones), and maintains a strict control of the protein-to-carbohydrate ratio at every meal.

Dr. Sears' eiconasoid-favorable diet could very well represent the future. Once we have more clinical support for this theory, I will certainly modify my present recommended ratio of 60 to 70 percent carbohydrates, 15 to 20 percent protein, and 15 to 20 percent fat. As I said before, nutrition is a tricky — and ever-evolving — field.

Appendix A

Illustrated Exercises

Caution
When working with free weights—especially barbells—you should
always have a spotter.

Chest Exercises

[a]:   [b]:

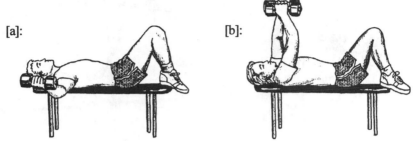

• *Flat Flye*. Lie flat on your back on the bench [a]. Holding a dumbbell in each hand, palms facing inward, slowly raise your arms straight up above your shoulders, keeping them slightly curved (as if you were hugging a tree) [b]. Slowly move the dumbbells apart and down, until you feel the stretch in your chest. Continue the exercise until you have completed the correct number of repetitions.

[a]:   [b]:

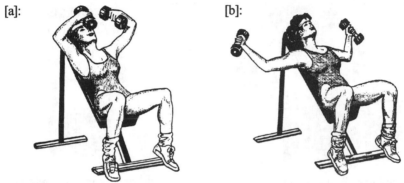

• *Incline Flye*. Keeping your back flat, position yourself on an incline bench. Holding a dumbbell in each hand, palms facing inward, slowly raise your arms straight up above your shoulders, keeping them slightly curved [a]. Slowly move the dumbbells apart and down until you feel the stretch in your chest [b]. Continue the exercise until you have completed the correct number of repetitions.

[a]:   [b]:

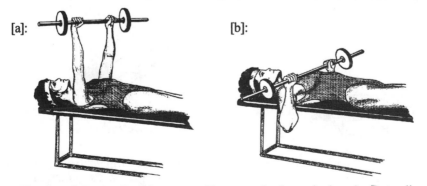

• *Flat Bench Press*. Position yourself on your back on the bench. Extending both arms straight, grasp the bar [a]. Slowly lower the weight to your chest [b], and then slowly return the bar to the starting position. Continue the exercise until you have completed the correct number of repetitions.

[a]:   [b]:

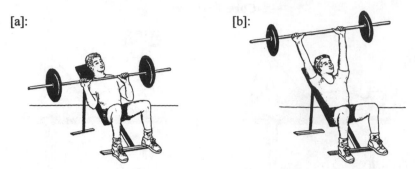

• *Incline Bench Press With Barbell.* Keeping your back flat, position yourself on an incline bench. Extending both arms straight, grasp the bar. Slowly lower the weight to your chest [a], and then slowly return the bar to the starting position [b]. Continue the exercise until you have completed the correct number of repetitions.

[a]:   [b]:

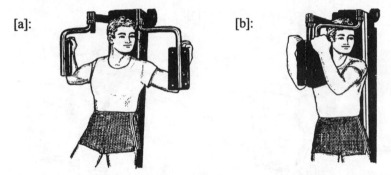

• *Pec Deck.* Position yourself at a pec deck machine with your forearms behind the pads, so that your arms and forearms are in front of the plane of your shoulders [a]. Slowly pull your forearms together until they are shoulder-width apart [b]. Hold for a second, and then slowly move your forearms back to the starting position. Continue the exercise until you have completed the correct number of repetitions.

[a]:   [b]:

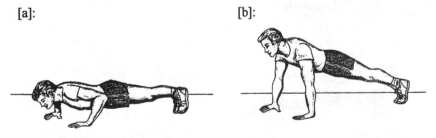

• *Push-Up.* Position yourself on the floor with your arms extended straight down below your shoulders, supporting your weight on the palms of your hands and balls of your feet. Bending your elbows, and holding your body rigid, slowly lower your chest to the floor [a]. Then slowly push yourself back up to the starting position [b]. Continue the exercise until you have completed the correct number of repetitions.

[a]: [b]:

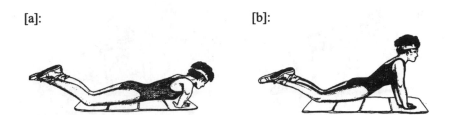

• *Modified Push-Up.* Position yourself on the floor with your arms extended straight down from your shoulders, supporting your weight on the palms of your hands and your knees. Bending your elbows, and holding your body rigid, slowly lower your chest to the floor [a]. Then slowly push yourself back up to the starting position [b]. Continue the exercise until you have completed the correct number of repetitions.

[a]: [b]:

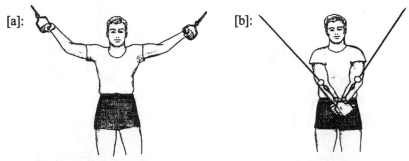

• *Cable Cross.* Position yourself at the crossover pulley machine with your feet slightly apart, your body bent slightly forward at the waist, and one pulley handle in each hand. Begin with your arms slightly bent, and held out and up at a 45-degree angle [a]. Slowly pull the handles down and forward until your wrists cross in front of you [b]. Hold for a second, and then slowly raise your arms to the starting position. Continue the exercise until you have completed the correct number of repetitions.

Back Exercises

[a]: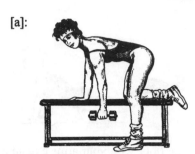

[b]: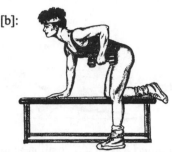

• *Bent Over Row With Dumbbell.* With your right hand and right knee, support yourself on the exercise bench. Holding a dumbbell in your left hand, let your left arm hang straight down [a]. Keeping your back straight, slowly pull the dumbbell upward towards your waist [b], and then slowly lower the weight to the starting position. Continue the exercise with your right arm until you have completed the correct number of repetitions, and then repeat the exercise with your left arm.

[a]: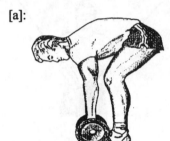

[b]: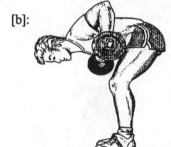

• *Bent Over Row With Barbell.* Stand behind the barbell with your feet flat on the floor shoulder-width apart, and your knees slightly bent. Bend over at the waist and grip the barbell just beyond shoulder width [a]. Slowly pull the weight up to your chest, bending your elbows [b]. Slowly lower the weight to the starting position, and continue the exercise until you have completed the correct number of repetitions.

[a]: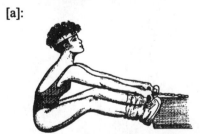

[b]: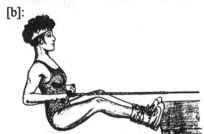

• *Seated Pulley Row.* Sit on the floor in front of the rowing machine with your legs slightly bent and your heels pressed firmly against the foot rest. Bending forward at the waist, extend your arms and grasp the pulley bar with an overhand grip [a]. Then pull the bar toward you as you straighten your back and pull yourself to an upright position [b]. Slowly return to the starting position, stretching forward as far as you can, and continue the exercise until you have completed the correct number of repetitions.

[a]:   [b]:

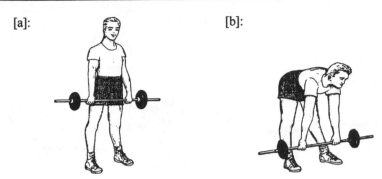

• *Stiff-Legged Deadlift*. Standing with your feet shoulder-width apart, hold a barbell down in front of your thighs [a]. Keeping your knees and back straight, slowly bend forward and lower the barbell until it touches the floor [b]. Then slowly straighten up, pulling the weight back to the starting position. Continue the exercise until you have completed the correct number of repetitions.

[a]:   [b]:

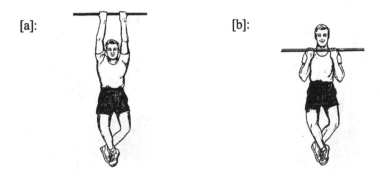

• *Pull-Up*. Grasp the bar securely with an underhand grip, and hang down as far as you can [a]. Slowly pull yourself up [b], and then slowly lower yourself back down to the starting position. Continue the exercise until you have completed the correct number of repetitions.

[a]:   [b]:

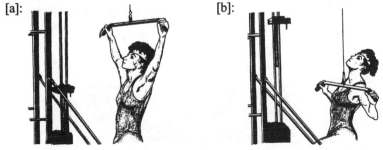

• *Lat Machine Pulldown to the Front*. Position yourself in the machine seat with your knees under the restraining bars. Grasp the bar with an overhand grip, palms facing forward [a]. Using your back muscles, slowly pull the bar down until it touches your upper chest [b]. Slowly return the bar to the starting position, and continue the exercise until you have completed the correct number of repetitions.

Abdominal Exercises

[a]:   [b]:

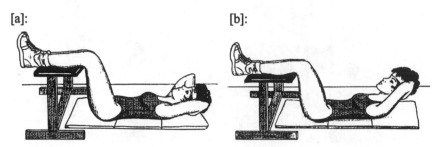

• *Abdominal Crunch With Bench.* Lie on the floor, flat on your back, in front of the exercise bench. Rest your lower legs on the bench, forming a 90 degree angle at the knee. Clasp your hands behind your neck [a], and use your abdominal and shoulder muscles to slowly raise your shoulders off the floor [b], and then slowly return to the starting position. Continue the exercise until you have completed the correct number of repetitions.

[a]:   [b]:

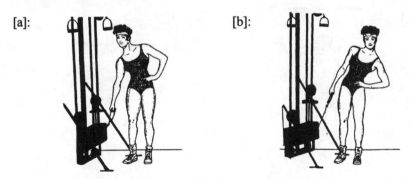

• *Oblique Crunch.* Position yourself with your right side next to the pulley machine, your feet slightly apart, and a pulley handle in your right hand [a]. Holding your left hand on your left hip, slowly bend away from the machine, keeping your right arm straight. Raise the pulley handle up to your thigh, making sure you feel the stretch on your right side and the crunch on your left side [b], and then slowly return to the starting position. Continue the exercise on your right side until you have completed the correct number of repetitions, and then repeat the exercise on your left side.

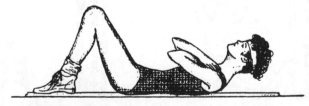

• *Bent-Knee Sit-Up.* Lie on the floor, flat on your back, with your knees bent and your arms folded across your chest. Using your abdominal muscles, slowly raise your head and shoulders until you are at a 30- to 45-degree angle to the floor, and then slowly lower yourself to the starting position. Continue the exercise until you have completed the correct number of repetitions.
(Note: DO NOT use a partner or a bench to stabilize your feet on the floor.)

[a]:   [b]:

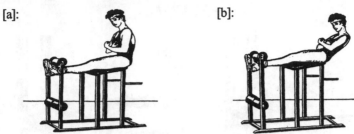

• *Roman Chair Sit-Up With Weights.* Position yourself on the Roman chair with your feet under the foot holder. Hold a light weight in each hand, crossing your arms over your chest [a]. Squeezing your abdominal muscles, slowly lower yourself until your body is almost parallel to the floor [b]. Then slowly return to the starting position. Continue the exercise until you have completed the correct number of repetitions.

Leg Exercises

[a]: [b]:

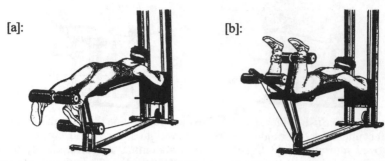

• *Leg Curl*. Lie on your stomach with your knees positioned at the end of the bench and your heels under the roller pads [a]. Flexing your hamstrings, slowly raise your feet until your legs form a 90-degree angle at the knee [b]. Hold for a second, and then slowly lower your legs to the starting position. Continue the exercise until you have completed the correct number of repetitions.

[a]: [b]:

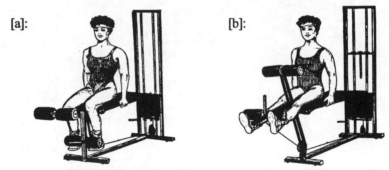

• *Leg Extension*. Position yourself in the machine seat with your ankles under the roller pads [a]. Flexing your quadriceps, slowly extend your legs out straight [b]. Hold for a second, and then slowly lower your legs to the starting position. Continue the exercise until you have completed the correct number of repetitions.

[a]: [b]:

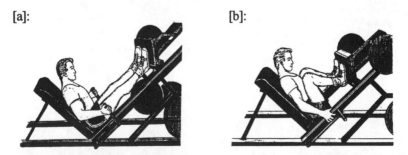

• *Leg Press*. Position yourself at the machine with your feet shoulder-width apart on the weighted platform, and your toes pointing slightly outward. Gripping the sides of the padded surface with your hands, slowly push the weight up until your legs are straight, but there is a slight bend at the knee [a]. Then slowly return to the starting position [b]. Continue the exercise until you have completed the correct numer of repetitions.

[a]: 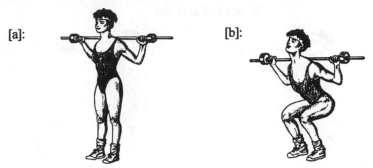 [b]:

• *Squat (Knee-Bend) With Barbell.* Resting a barbell behind your neck, stand with your feet shoulder-width apart [a]. Keeping your head and back straight, slowly bend at the knees and lower yourself into a squatting position [b]. Go as far as you can without putting too much strain on your knees, and then slowly raise yourself up to the starting position. Continue the exercise until you have completed the correct number of repetitions.

[a]: 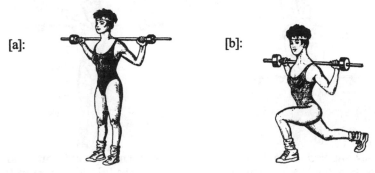 [b]:

• *Leg Lunge With Barbell.* Holding a barbell behind your neck, stand with your feet about 6 inches apart [a]. Keeping your head and back straight, step forward with your left leg, bending until the knee of your right leg almost touches the floor [b]. Then slowly raise yourself up to the starting position, and repeat with the right leg. Continue the exercise until you have completed the correct number of repetitions.

Shoulder Exercises

[a]: 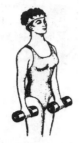 [b]: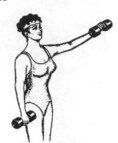

• *Front Raise With Dumbbells.* Standing with your feet shoulder-width apart, hold a dumbbell in each hand, and let your arms hang straight down in front of your thighs [a]. Without bending your elbows, slowly raise your right arm to above shoulder height. Then slowly lower your right arm to the rest position before raising your left arm to above shoulder height [b]. Continue alternating arms until you have completed the correct number of repetitions.

[a]: 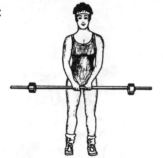   [b]: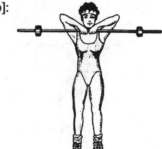

• *Upright Row With Barbell or Dumbbells.* Using an overhand grip, hold a barbell or two dumbbells down in front of your thighs [a]. Slowly raise the weight to your chin, keeping your elbows up [b]. Flex your shoulders, and then slowly lower the weight to the starting position. Continue the exercise until you have completed the correct number of repetitions.

[a]: 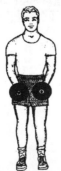 [b]: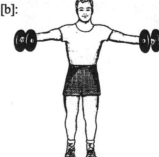

• *Lateral Raise.* Standing with your feet shoulder-width apart, hold a dumbbell in each hand, and let your hands hang down at your sides with your palms facing in [a]. Without bending your elbows, slowly raise your arms to above the shoulder or eye level [b]. Then slowly lower the weights to the starting position. Continue the exercise until you have completed the correct number of repetitions.

[a]: 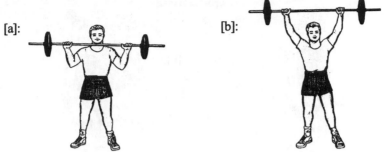 [b]:

• *Shoulder Press.* Resting a barbell across your shoulders and chest, stand with your feet shoulder-width apart [a]. Keeping your head and back straight, slowly raise the weight until your arms are fully extended [b]. Hold for a second, and then slowly lower the weight to the starting position. Continue the exercise until you have completed the correct number of repetitions.

Triceps Exercises

[a]: 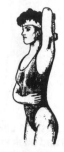   [b]: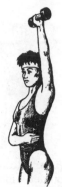

• *One-Arm Dumbbell Triceps Curl.* Hold a dumbbell in your left hand, behind your neck [a]. Slowly raise the weight straight up until your arm is fully extended, keeping the arm close to the side of your head [b]. Then, slowly lower the weight to the starting position. Continue the exercise with your left arm until you have completed the correct number of repetitions, and then repeat the exercise with your right arm.

[a]: 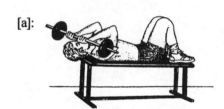   [b]: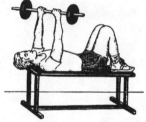

• *Lying Triceps Extension.* Position yourself on your back with your knees bent up and your feet on the bench. Hold the barbell above your forehead, with your arms bent and your hands about seven inches apart [a]. Slowly extend your arms straight up [b], and then slowly lower the weight to the starting position. Continue the exercise until you have completed the correct number of repetitions.

[a]: 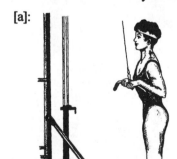   [b]: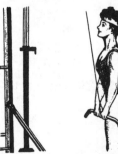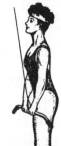

• *Cable Pressdown.* Face the machine and grasp the bar with an overhand grip. Position your hands about 6 inches apart. Keeping your upper arms close to your body, bend at the elbows, and extend your forearms upward [a]. Then slowly push down on the bar until your arms are completely straight [b]. Slowly return the bar to the starting position, and continue the exercises until you have completed the correct number of repetitions. You may use a short bar or triceps bar if available.

Biceps Exercises

[a]: 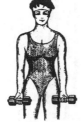 [b]: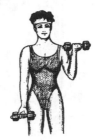

• *Alternate-Arm Standing Dumbbell Curl.* Standing with your feet shoulder-width apart, hold a dumbbell in each hand, and let your arms hang straight down close to your sides [a]. Bending at the elbow, slowly raise your right arm to shoulder height. Then slowly lower your right arm to the rest position before raising your left arm [b]. Continue alternating arms until you have completed the correct number of repetitions.

[a]: 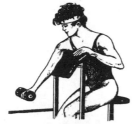 [b]: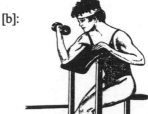

• *One-Arm Preacher Curl.* Position yourself at the preacher bench with the edge of the bench supporting your body under your right armpit. Holding a dumbbell in your right hand, lean forward and let your right arm hang straight down, keeping your wrist straight [a]. Raise the dumbbell until it touches your chin [b]. Then slowly lower the dumbbell to the starting position. Continue the exercise with your right arm until you have completed the correct number of repetitions, and then repeat the exercise with your left arm.

[a]: 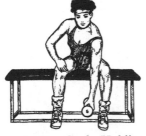 [b]: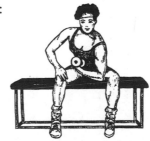

• *Concentration Curl.* Holding a dumbbell in your left hand, sit on a flat exercise bench with your feet approximately two feet apart. Bending forward at the waist, rest your left elbow on your left thigh, letting your left arm hang straight down towards the floor [a]. Keeping your wrist straight, slowly pull the dumbbell towards your chest until your elbow is completely bent [b], and then slowly lower the dumbbell to the starting position. Continue the exercise with your left arm until you have completed the correct number of repetitions, and then repeat the exercise with your right arm.

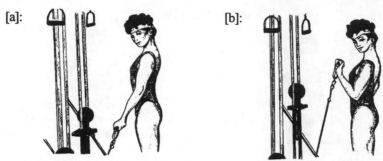

• *Pulley Curl.* Face the pulley machine with your feet shoulder-width apart and your arms straight at your sides. Relax your right arm and grasp the pulley handle with your left hand, palm up [a]. Flexing your biceps, slowly raise your left forearm until it is fully flexed [b]. Then slowly return to the starting position. Continue the exercise with your left arm until you have completed the correct number of repetitions, and then repeat the exercise with your right arm.

Beginner
Exercise Program

Note

The programs suggested on the following pages represent merely a sampling of the many exercises you can do to strengthen specific muscle groups. Consult a weight-training professional for further recommendations.

<u>Choose 2 Exercises</u>:
- *Flat Flye*   • *Incline Flye*
- *Flat Bench Press*
• *Incline Bench Press With Barbell*   • *Pec Deck*
• *Push-Up (for men) or Modified Push-Up (for women)*

	Weeks 1 & 2	Weeks 3 & 4	Weeks 5 & 6	Weeks 7 & 8	Weeks 9 & 10	Weeks 11 & 12
Recommended Weight *(As % of maximum weight for 1 rep)*	50%	50%	60%	70%	80%	**Pyramids (Start at 70% for set 1, and increase for sets 2 and 3.)
Number of Sets	1	2	3	3	3	3
Repetitions	10-12	10-12	10-12	8-10	8-10	set 1 = 10 set 2 = 6-8 set 3 = 4-6
Rest Period Between Reps	60-90 secs.	60-90 secs.	60-90 secs.	60-90 secs.	60-90 secs.	2 mins.
Frequency	M-W-F	M-W-F	M-W-F	M-W-F	M-W-F	M-W-F

*For example, if the maximum weight you can lift for 1 rep is 100 lbs. —
for weeks 1 - 4 you will lift 50% of that, or 50 lbs.;
for weeks 5 & 6 you will lift 60% of that, or 60 lbs., etc.
**See page 127 for definition of a "pyramid."*

Beginner Program — Back

<u>**Choose 2 Exercises**</u>:
- *Bent-Over Row With Dumbbell*   • *Bent-Over Row With Barbell*
- *Seated Pulley Row*
- *Stiff-Legged Deadlift*   • *Pull-Up*
- *Lat-Machine Pulldown to the Front*

	Weeks 1 & 2	Weeks 3 & 4	Weeks 5 & 6	Weeks 7 & 8	Weeks 9 & 10	Weeks 11 & 12
Recommended Weight *(As % of maximum weight for 1 rep)*	50%	50%	60%	70%	80%	**Pyramids (Start at 70% for set 1, and increase for sets 2 and 3.)
Number of Sets	1	2	3	3	3	3
Repetitions	10-12	10-12	10-12	10-12	10-12	set 1 = 10 set 2 = 6-8 set 3 = 4-6
Rest Period Between Reps	60-90 secs.	60-90 secs.	60-90 secs.	60-90 secs.	60-90 secs.	2 mins.
Frequency	M-W-F	M-W- F	M-W-F	M-W-F	M-W-F	M-W-F

For example, if the maximum weight you can lift for 1 rep is 100 lbs. —
for weeks 1 - 4 you will lift 50% of that, or 50 lbs.;
for weeks 5 & 6 you will lift 60% of that, or 60 lbs., etc.
**See page 127 for definition of a "pyramid."*

Beginner Program — Abdomen

<u>Choose 2 Exercises</u>:
* *Abdominal Crunch With Bench*
* *Oblique Crunch*
* *Bent-Knee Sit-Up*
* *Roman Chair Sit-Up With Weights*

	Weeks 1 & 2	Weeks 3 & 4	Weeks 5 & 6	Weeks 7 & 8	Weeks 9 & 10	Weeks 11 & 12
Number of Sets	1	2	3	3	3	3
Repetitions	10-20	10-20	10-20	20 or more	30 or more	30 or more
Rest Period Between Reps	60-90 secs.	60-90 secs.	60-90 secs.	60-90 secs.	60-90 secs.	30 secs.
Frequency	M-W-F	M-W- F	M-W-F	M-W-F	M-W-F	M-W-F

Choose 1 Exercise From Each Group:

A
• Leg Curl
• Leg Lunge With Barbell

B
• Leg Extension
• Leg Press
• Squat (Knee-Bend) With Barbell

	Weeks 1 & 2	Weeks 3 & 4	Weeks 5 & 6	Weeks 7 & 8	Weeks 9 & 10	Weeks 11 & 12
Recommended Weight *(As % of maximum weight for 1 rep)*	50%	50%	60%	70%	80%	**Pyramids (Start at 70% for set 1, and increase for sets 2 and 3.)
Number of Sets	1	2	3	3	3	3
Repetitions	15-20	15-20	15-20	10-12	10-12	set 1 = 10 set 2 = 6-8 set 3 = 4-6
Rest Period Between Reps	60-90 secs.	60-90 secs.	60-90 secs.	60-90 secs.	60-90 secs.	2 mins.
Frequency	M-W-F	M-W- F	M-W-F	M-W-F	M-W-F	M-W-F

*For example, if the maximum weight you can lift for 1 rep is 100 lbs. —
for weeks 1 - 4 you will lift 50% of that, or 50 lbs.;
for weeks 5 & 6 you will lift 60% of that, or 60 lbs., etc.
**See page 127 for definition of a "pyramid."

Beginner Program — Shoulders

Choose 1 Exercise:
- *Front Raise With Dumbbells*
- *Upright Row With Barbell or Dumbbells*
- *Lateral Raise*

	Weeks 1 & 2	Weeks 3 & 4	Weeks 5 & 6	Weeks 7 & 8	Weeks 9 & 10	Weeks 11 & 12
Recommended Weight *(As % of maximum weight for 1 rep)*	50%	50%	60%	70%	80%	**Pyramids (Start at 70% for set 1, and increase for sets 2 and 3.)
Number of Sets	1	2	3	3	3	3
Repetitions	10-12	10-12	10-12	10-12	10-12	set 1 = 10 set 2 = 6-8 set 3 = 4-6
Rest Period Between Reps	60-90 secs.	60-90 secs.	60-90 secs.	60-90 secs.	60-90 secs.	2 mins.
Frequency	M-W-F	M-W- F	M-W-F	M-W-F	M-W-F	M-W-F

*For example, if the maximum weight you can lift for 1 rep is 100 lbs. —
for weeks 1 - 4 you will lift 50% of that, or 50 lbs.;
for weeks 5 & 6 you will lift 60% of that, or 60 lbs., etc.
**See page 127 for definition of a "pyramid."

Beginner Program — Triceps

Choose 1 Exercise:
• One-Arm Dumbbell Triceps Curl
• Lying Triceps Extension
• Cable Pressdown

	Weeks 1 & 2	Weeks 3 & 4	Weeks 5 & 6	Weeks 7 & 8	Weeks 9 & 10	Weeks 11 & 12
Recommended Weight *(As % of maximum weight for 1 rep)*	50%	50%	60%	70%	80%	**Pyramids (Start at 70% for set 1, and increase for sets 2 and 3.)
Number of Sets	1	2	3	3	3	3
Repetitions	10-12	10-12	10-12	10-12	10-12	set 1 = 10 set 2 = 6-8 set 3 = 4-6
Rest Period Between Reps	60-90 secs.	60-90 secs.	60-90 secs.	60-90 secs.	60-90 secs.	2 mins.
Frequency	M-W-F	M-W- F	M-W-F	M-W-F	M-W-F	M-W-F

For example, if the maximum weight you can lift for 1 rep is 100 lbs. —
for weeks 1 - 4 you will lift 50% of that, or 50 lbs.;
for weeks 5 & 6 you will lift 60% of that, or 60 lbs., etc.
***See page 127 for definition of a "pyramid."*

Beginner Program — Biceps

Choose 1 Exercise:
• *Alternate-Arm Standing Dumbbell Curl*
• *One-Arm Preacher Curl*
• *Concentration Curl*
• *Pulley Curl*

	Weeks 1 & 2	Weeks 3 & 4	Weeks 5 & 6	Weeks 7 & 8	Weeks 9 & 10	Weeks 11 & 12
Recommended Weight *(As % of maximum weight for 1 rep)*	50%	50%	60%	70%	80%	**Pyramids (Start at 70% for set 1, and increase for sets 2 and 3.)
Number of Sets	1	2	3	3	3	3
Repetitions	10-12	10-12	10-12	10-12	10-12	set 1 = 10 set 2 = 6-8 set 3 = 4-6
Rest Period Between Reps	60-90 secs.	60-90 secs.	60-90 secs.	60-90 secs.	60-90 secs.	2 mins.
Frequency	M-W-F	M-W- F	M-W-F	M-W-F	M-W-F	M-W-F

*For example, if the maximum weight you can lift for 1 rep is 100 lbs. —
for weeks 1 - 4 you will lift 50% of that, or 50 lbs.;
for weeks 5 & 6 you will lift 60% of that, or 60 lbs., etc.
**See page 127 for definition of a "pyramid."

Appendix C

Intermediate Exercise Program

> **Note**
> The programs suggested on the following pages represent merely a sampling of the many exercises you can do to strengthen specific muscle groups. Consult a weight-training professional for further recommendations.

Intermediate Program — Chest

Choose 1 Exercise From Each Group:

A
- Flat Flye
- Flat Bench Press

B
- Incline Flye
- Incline Bench Press With Barbell

C
- Pec Deck
- Push-Up
- Cable Cross

	Weeks 1 - 4	Weeks 5 - 8	Weeks 9 - 12
Recommended Weight *(As % of maximum weight for 1 rep)*	**Pyramids (70% - 80% - 90%) Per Exercise	**Pyramids (70% - 80% - 90%) Per Exercise	**Pyramids (70% - 80% - 90%) Per Exercise
Number of Sets	3	3	4
Repetitions	set 1 = 10 set 2 = 6-8 set 3 = 4-6	set 1 = 10 set 2 = 6-8 set 3 = 4-6	set 1 = 10 set 2 = 6-8 set 3 = 4-6 set 4 = 4-6
Rest Period Between Reps	2-3 mins.	2-3 mins.	2-3 mins.
Frequency	M-W-F	M-Th	M-Th

*For example, if the maximum weight you can lift for 1 rep is 100 lbs. —
for set 1 you will lift 70% of that, or 70 lbs.;
for set 2 you will lift 80% of that, or 80 lbs., etc.
**See page 127 for definition of a "pyramid."

Choose 1 Exercise From Each Group:

A
- *Bent-Over Row With Dumbbell*
- *Bent-Over Row With Barbell*

B   ### C
- *Seated Pulley Row*   • *Stiff-Legged Deadlift*
- *Pull-Up*
- *Lat-Machine Pulldown to the Front*

	Weeks 1 - 4	Weeks 5 - 8	Weeks 9 - 12
Recommended Weight *(As % of maximum weight for 1 rep)*	**Pyramids (70% - 80% - 90%) Per Exercise	**Pyramids (70% - 80% - 90%) Per Exercise	**Pyramids (70% - 80% - 90%) Per Exercise
Number of Sets	3	3	4
Repetitions	set 1 = 10 set 2 = 6-8 set 3 = 4-6	set 1 = 10 set 2 = 6-8 set 3 = 4-6	set 1 = 10 set 2 = 6-8 set 3 = 4-6 set 4 = 4-6
Rest Period Between Reps	2-3 mins.	2-3 mins.	2-3 mins.
Frequency	M-W-F	Tu-F	Tu-F

*For example, if the maximum weight you can lift for 1 rep is 100 lbs. —
for set 1 you will lift 70% of that, or 70 lbs.;
for set 2 you will lift 80% of that, or 80 lbs., etc.
**See page 127 for definition of a "pyramid."

Intermediate Program — Abdomen

Choose 1 Exercise From Each Group:

A
• *Abdominal Crunch With Bench With Weights*
B   *C*
• *Bent-Knee Sit-Up With Weights*   • *Oblique Crunch*
                                           • *Roman Chair Sit-Up With Weights*

	Weeks 1 - 4	Weeks 5 - 8	Weeks 9 - 12
Recommended Weight *(As % of maximum weight for 1 rep)*	**Pyramids (70% - 80% - 90%) Per Exercise	**Pyramids (70% - 80% - 90%) Per Exercise	**Pyramids (70% - 80% - 90%) Per Exercise
Number of Sets	3	3	4
Repetitions	set 1 = 30 set 2 = 20-30 set 3 = 10-20	set 1 = 30 set 2 = 20-30 set 3 = 10-20	set 1 = 30 set 2 = 30 set 3 = 20 set 4 = 20
Rest Period Between Reps	1 min. or less	1 min. or less	1 min. or less
Frequency	Daily	Daily	Daily

For example, if the maximum weight you can lift for 1 rep is 100 lbs. —
for set 1 you will lift 70% of that, or 70 lbs.;
for set 2 you will lift 80% of that, or 80 lbs., etc.
***See page 127 for definition of a "pyramid."*

Intermediate Program — Legs

<u>**Choose 1 Exercise From Each Group**</u>:

A
* *Leg Extension*
* *Leg Press*

B   *C*
* *Squat (Knee-Bend) With Barbell*   * *Leg Curl*
                                         * *Leg Lunge With Barbell*

	Weeks 1 - 4	Weeks 5 - 8	Weeks 9 - 12
Recommended Weight *(As % of maximum weight for 1 rep)*	**Pyramids (70% - 80% - 90%) Per Exercise	**Pyramids (70% - 80% - 90%) Per Exercise	**Pyramids (70% - 80% - 90%) Per Exercise
Number of Sets	3	3	4
Repetitions	set 1 = 10 set 2 = 6-8 set 3 = 4-6	set 1 = 10 set 2 = 6-8 set 3 = 4-6	set 1 = 10 set 2 = 6-8 set 3 = 4-6 set 4 = 4-6
Rest Period Between Reps	2-3 mins.	2-3 mins.	2-3 mins.
Frequency	M-W-F	M-Th	M-Th

For example, if the maximum weight you can lift for 1 rep is 100 lbs. —
for set 1 you will lift 70% of that, or 70 lbs.;
for set 2 you will lift 80% of that, or 80 lbs., etc.
***See page 127 for definition of a "pyramid."*

Intermediate Program — Shoulders

Choose 1 Exercise From Each Group:

A	*B*
• Front Raise With Dumbbells	• Shoulder Press
• Lateral Raise	• Upright Row With Barbell or Dumbbells

	Weeks 1 - 4	Weeks 5 - 8	Weeks 9 - 12
Recommended Weight *(As % of maximum weight for 1 rep)*	**Pyramids (70% - 80% - 90%) Per Exercise	**Pyramids (70% - 80% - 90%) Per Exercise	**Pyramids (70% - 80% - 90%) Per Exercise
Number of Sets	3	3	4
Repetitions	set 1 = 10 set 2 = 6-8 set 3 = 4-6	set 1 = 10 set 2 = 6-8 set 3 = 4-6	set 1 = 10 set 2 = 6-8 set 3 = 4-6 set 4 = 4-6
Rest Period Between Reps	2-3 mins.	2-3 mins.	2-3 mins.
Frequency	M-W-F	M-Th	M-Th

*For example, if the maximum weight you can lift for 1 rep is 100 lbs. —
for set 1 you will lift 70% of that, or 70 lbs.;
for set 2 you will lift 80% of that, or 80 lbs., etc.
**See page 127 for definition of a "pyramid."

Intermediate Program — Triceps

Choose 1 Exercise From Each Group:

A	B
• One-Arm Dumbbell Triceps Curl	• Lying Triceps Extension
• Cable Pressdown	

	Weeks 1 - 4	Weeks 5 - 8	Weeks 9 - 12
Recommended Weight *(As % of maximum weight for 1 rep)*	**Pyramids (70% - 80% - 90%) Per Exercise	**Pyramids (70% - 80% - 90%) Per Exercise	**Pyramids (70% - 80% - 90%) Per Exercise
Number of Sets	3	3	4
Repetitions	set 1 = 10 set 2 = 6-8 set 3 = 4-6	set 1 = 10 set 2 = 6-8 set 3 = 4-6	set 1 = 10 set 2 = 6-8 set 3 = 4-6 set 4 = 4-6
Rest Period Between Reps	2-3 mins.	2-3 mins.	2-3 mins.
Frequency	M-W-F	M-Th	M-Th

*For example, if the maximum weight you can lift for 1 rep is 100 lbs. —
for set 1 you will lift 70% of that, or 70 lbs.;
for set 2 you will lift 80% of that, or 80 lbs., etc.
**See page 127 for definition of a "pyramid."

Intermediate Program — Biceps

Choose 1 Exercise From Each Group:
A
- *Alternate-Arm Standing Dumbbell Curl*
- *Pulley Curl*

B
- *One-Arm Preacher Curl*
- *Concentration Curl*

	Weeks 1 - 4	Weeks 5 - 8	Weeks 9 - 12
Recommended Weight *(As % of maximum weight for 1 rep)*	**Pyramids (70% - 80% - 90%) Per Exercise	**Pyramids (70% - 80% - 90%) Per Exercise	**Pyramids (70% - 80% - 90%) Per Exercise
Number of Sets	3	3	4
Repetitions	set 1 = 10 set 2 = 6-8 set 3 = 4-6	set 1 = 10 set 2 = 6-8 set 3 = 4-6	set 1 = 10 set 2 = 6-8 set 3 = 4-6 set 4 = 4-6
Rest Period Between Reps	2-3 mins.	2-3 mins.	2-3 mins.
Frequency	M-W-F	Tu-F	Tu-F

*For example, if the maximum weight you can lift for 1 rep is 100 lbs. —
for set 1 you will lift 70% of that, or 70 lbs.;
for set 2 you will lift 80% of that, or 80 lbs., etc.
**See page 127 for definition of a "pyramid."

Appendix D

Healthy Menus

Vegetarian Day 1

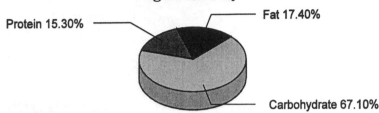

Protein 15.30%

Fat 17.40%

Carbohydrate 67.10%

BREAKFAST
1/2 grapefruit
1 cup hot oatmeal with:
    1 tablespoon honey
    1 tablespoon raisins
    1/4 cup dried dates pitted and chopped
    1 oz. chopped walnuts
    1/2 green apple cored and chopped
1 slice whole wheat toast
1 tablespoon orange marmalade
8 oz. skim milk
6 oz. hot beverage

LUNCH
5 oz. spicy vegetarian chili with beans
2 toasted corn tortillas
1 oz. salsa
Spinach salad:
    1 cup chopped raw spinach
    1/4 cup sliced raw mushrooms
    1 oz. part-skim mozzarella cheese
    1 tablespoon oil-free vinegar dressing
1 fresh peach

DINNER
Tofu-vegetable stir fry:
    1/2 cup carrots
    1/2 cup Chinese cabbage
    1/2 cup bamboo shoots
    1 spear broccoli
    1 piece tofu (2-1/2" x 2-3/4" x 1") cubed
3/4 cup brown rice with:
    1/8 cup chopped water chestnuts
    1/2 teaspoon ginger
Cucumber-tomato salad:
    3 large slices cucumber
    2 tomato wedges
    1 tablespoon oil-free vinegar dressing
1 pita bread
1 cup lowfat frozen yogurt

Vegetarian Day 2

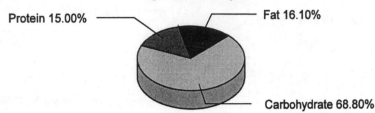

Protein 15.00%   Fat 16.10%

Carbohydrate 68.80%

BREAKFAST
2/3 cup shredded wheat with:
    1/2 cup blueberries
    1 tablespoon brown sugar
    8 oz. skim milk
1 slice raisin walnut bread
8 oz. apple juice
6 oz. hot beverage

LUNCH
Baked potato with:
    1/3 cup lowfat (less than 1%) cottage cheese
    1 teaspoon chives
1 cup French-style green beans with:
    1/2 oz. slivered almonds
    1 tablespoon lemon juice
1 pita bread
1 cup watermelon chunks

DINNER
1 cup cooked spaghetti with:
    1/2 cup fresh tomato and basil sauce
    1/2 cup eggplant
    1 oz. grated Parmesan cheese
    1/4 oz. pine nuts
Chicory and alfalfa salad:
    1 cup chopped chicory
    1/2 cup alfalfa sprouts
    1/8 cup thinly sliced mushrooms
    1/8 red pepper deseeded and sliced
    1 tablespoon chopped onion
    1 tablespoon oil-free vinegar dressing
2 flatbread crackers
1 cinnamon baked apple

Vegetarian Day 3

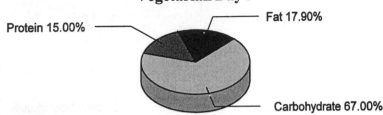

Protein 15.00%

Fat 17.90%

Carbohydrate 67.00%

BREAKFAST
1/2 cantaloupe
1/4 cup scrambled egg substitute with:
    1/4 cup mushrooms
    1 oz. cheddar cheese shredded
    1 tablespoon chives
1 toasted pita bread
8 oz. orange juice
6 oz. hot beverage

LUNCH
Belgian endive salad:
    1 cup Belgian endive finely sliced
    1/2 cup Chinese cabbage leaves shredded
    1/2 cup grapefruit sections
    1/4 cup sweet orange slices
    1/4 cup golden raisins
    1/3 cup chickpeas
    1/2 oz. chopped walnuts
    1-1/2 tablespoons orange/lemon/honey dressing
1 slice cracked wheat bread toasted
6 oz. fruit-flavored nonfat yogurt

DINNER
Stuffed pepper:
    1 large red or yellow pepper cored and deseeded
    1/3 cup bread stuffing
    1/8 cup dried apricots
    1 tablespoon chopped onion
    1 oz. plain nonfat yogurt
3/4 cup white rice
3/4 cup lima beans mixed with 1/4 cup diced zucchini
1 slice flatbread
1 cup diced pineapple with:
    1/3 cup lowfat (less than 1%) cottage cheese
    1/2 oz. filberts (hazelnuts) sliced and toasted

Vegetarian Day 4

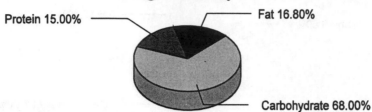

Protein 15.00% — Fat 16.80%

Carbohydrate 68.00%

BREAKFAST
Banana yogurt smoothie:
    1 cup sliced banana
    6 oz. lowfat strawberry yogurt
    4 oz. apple juice
1 whole wheat bagel
1-1/2 tablespoons peanut butter
6 oz. hot beverage

LUNCH
7-1/2 oz. split pea soup
1 corn on the cob
1 pita bread toasted
1 cup fresh berries
1/2 oz. Brazil nuts shelled

DINNER
Veggie soft tacos:
    2 flour tortillas
    3/4 cup refried beans
    1/4 shredded lettuce
    1/4 cup diced tomato
    1/4 cup sliced squash
    1 oz. lowfat cheddar cheese
    1 tablespoon peppers
    1 tablespoon onion
    2 tablespoons salsa
Cole slaw:
    3/4 cup shredded cabbage
    1/4 cup shredded carrots
    1 oz. lowfat yogurt
    1 tablespoon lemon juice
    1 tablespoon honey
1/2 cup light vanilla ice milk with:
    10 sweet pitted cherries
    1 tablespoon oat-bran flakes

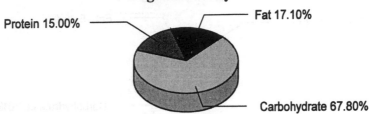

Vegetarian Day 5

Protein 15.00% — Fat 17.10% — Carbohydrate 67.80%

BREAKFAST
1 cup sliced orange
French toast:
    1 slice whole wheat bread
    1/4 cup egg substitute
    1 tablespoon skim milk
    1/4 teaspoon cinnamon
    1/2 oz. chopped walnuts
    1/2 cup sliced strawberries
    1/2 teaspoon powdered sugar
8 oz. pineapple juice
6 oz. hot beverage

LUNCH
Navy bean salad:
    1 cup boiled navy beans
    1/4 red pepper cored, deseeded, and thinly sliced
    1 leek thinly sliced
    1 scallion thinly sliced
    1/2 teaspoon French-style mustard
    2 teaspoons olive oil
    1 tablespoon red wine vinegar
1 pita bread with 1/2 cup chickpea spread
1 kiwi

DINNER
Vegetable curry:
    1/4 cup squash
    1/4 cup mushroom
    1/4 cup carrots
    1/4 cup red pepper
    1/2 teaspoon curry
    1/2 teaspoon other seasonings
3/4 cup cooked pasta
1/2 cup lowfat (less than 1%) cottage cheese
1 slice flatbread
Apricot crumble:
    1 cup diced apricots in juice
    1-1/2 tablespoons golden raisins
    1/4 oz. granola
    1/2 oz. chopped almonds
    1 tablespoon honey
    1/4 teaspoon ginger

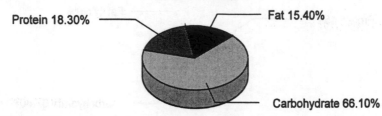

Vegetarian Day 6

Protein 18.30% —

Fat 15.40%

Carbohydrate 66.10%

BREAKFAST
1/2 honeydew melon
1 toasted English muffin
1 tablespoon fruit spread
1/2 oz. pecan halves
8 oz. skim milk
6 oz. hot beverage

LUNCH
Vegetable pita pizza:
    1 pita bread
    1/4 cup braised eggplant
    1/4 cup sliced mushrooms
    1 tablespoon green or red pepper
    1 tablespoon onion
    1/4 teaspoon fresh garlic
    2 tablespoons tomato sauce
    1 oz. part-skim mozzarella cheese
Mixed green salad:
    1 cup spinach
    1/2 cup radiccio
    1/4 cup sliced beets
    1 tablespoon nonfat dressing
4 oz. tapioca pudding topped with shredded coconut

DINNER
1 cup mixed beans (pinto, lima, kidney, black-eyed peas)
1 cup white rice
1 cup steamed zucchini squash with:
    1/4 cup stewed tomatoes
    1 tablespoon olive oil
    1/4 teaspoon minced garlic
1 multi-grain roll
1 cup applesauce

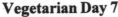

Vegetarian Day 7

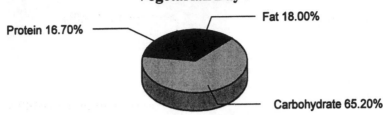

Protein 16.70%

Fat 18.00%

Carbohydrate 65.20%

BREAKFAST
1 cup fresh strawberries
1 cup cream of wheat with:
     1-1/2 tablespoons raisins
     1/2 oz. slivered almonds
     1/2 teaspoon cinnamon
1 slice multi-grain toast
1 tablespoon fruit spread
8 oz. skim milk
6 oz. hot beverage

LUNCH
9.5 oz. lentil soup
Apple-celery salad:
     3/4 cup sliced apple
     1/4 cup chopped celery
     1/4 oz. chopped walnuts
     1 cup lettuce
Dressing of:
     1 tablespoon lowfat yogurt
     1 tablespoon honey
     1 tablespoon lime juice
1 slice flatbread
1 oz. part-skim cheddar cheese
1/2 cup fruit-flavored gelatin

DINNER
Manicotti:
     2 manicotti shells
     2 oz. tofu
     1 cup part-skim ricotta
     1 oz. tomato sauce
     1 teaspoon Italian seasoning
1 cup steamed broccoli and cauliflower with lemon juice and seasoning
Tossed salad:
     3/4 cup lettuce
     1/4 cup red cabbage
     1/4 cup carrots
     1/8 cup sweet peppers
     1 tablespoon nonfat dressing
1 pita bread
10 seedless grapes

Semi-Vegetarian Day 1

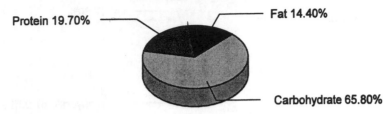

Protein 19.70% — Fat 14.40%

Carbohydrate 65.80%

BREAKFAST
1/2 grapefruit
1 oz. oat-bran granola with:
    1/2 cup blueberries
    8 oz. skim milk
1 slice whole wheat toast
8 oz. orange juice
6 oz. hot beverage

LUNCH
9.5 oz. Italian vegetable pasta soup
Pita sandwich:
    1 pita bread
    3/4 cup chickpea spread
    1/2 cup lettuce
    3 slices cucumber
    1 tablespoon chopped onion
1 medium apple
1.5 oz. part-skim cheddar cheese

DINNER
3 oz. skinless lemon-roasted chicken breast
3/4 cup baked rice with:
    1/2 cup mushrooms
    1 tablespoon scallions
4 spears steamed asparagus with lemon juice
Mixed salad:
    1 cup lettuce
    1/4 green pepper sliced
    1 spear broccoli chopped
    1 tablespoon nonfat red wine vinaigrette
1 piece flatbread
1 cup oranges simmered with:
    1/2 oz. chopped cashews
    1 tablespoon honey
    1 teaspoon cinnamon
    1/2 teaspoon ginger

Semi-Vegetarian Day 2

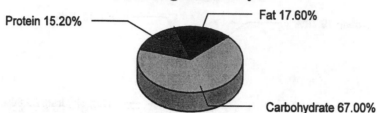

Protein 15.20% — Fat 17.60%

Carbohydrate 67.00%

BREAKFAST
1/2 cantaloupe
1 cup hot oatmeal with:
    1 tablespoon honey
    1 tablespoon golden raisins
    1/4 cup dried dates pitted and chopped
    1 oz. chopped walnuts
    1/2 green apple cored and chopped
1 slice whole wheat toast
1 tablespoon strawberry preserves
8 oz. skim milk
6 oz. hot beverage

LUNCH
Tuna sandwich:
    2 slices whole wheat bread
    2 ounces white tuna (in water)
    1 teaspoon chopped onion
    1 tablespoon chopped celery
    1 tablespoon lowfat yogurt
    1 teaspoon dijon mustard
    1 teaspoon honey
    1/2 cup lettuce
    2 tomato slices
3/4 cup steamed peas and carrots
1 medium-sized pear

DINNER
Spinach/mushroom lasagne:
    1 cup pasta
    1/2 cup spinach
    1/4 cup sliced mushrooms
    1/4 cup part-skim ricotta
    1 oz. part-skim mozzarella
    1/3 cup mushroom marinara sauce
1 slice multi-grain bread
Tossed salad:
    1 cup lettuce
    1 tablespoon chopped onion
    1/4 cup sliced beets
    1 tablespoon nonfat dressing
1 cup 2% sherbert

Semi-Vegetarian Day 3

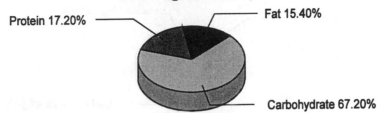

Protein 17.20% — Fat 15.40%

Carbohydrate 67.20%

BREAKFAST
1 cup fruit salad (watermelon, strawberries, cantaloupe, and honeydew)
1 whole wheat bagel
1/4 cup lowfat cottage cheese
1 oz. smoked salmon
8 oz. grapefruit juice
6 oz. hot beverage

LUNCH
7.5 oz. chunky 5-bean soup
Spinach-stuffed tomato:
      1 tomato
      1/2 cup cooked spinach
      1 tablespoon plain lowfat yogurt
      1 tablespoon breadcrumbs
      1/2 oz. grated Parmesan cheese
1 slice flatbread
Carrot sticks/pepper rings
1 nectarine

DINNER
Scallop kebabs:
      6 scallops marinated in orange juice, lemon juice, and garlic
      3/4 cup zucchini
      1/4 cup red onion
1 baked sweet potato
Healthy coleslaw:
      1/2 cup cabbage
      1/4 cup carrots
      1 tablespoon plain lowfat yogurt
      1 teaspoon honey
      1 tablespoon apple cider vinegar
1 multi-grain roll
1/2 cup lowfat frozen yogurt topped with cherries

Semi-Vegetarian Day 4

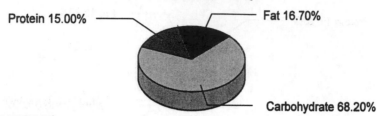

Protein 15.00% — Fat 16.70%

Carbohydrate 68.20%

BREAKFAST
1 cup sliced peaches
French toast:
  1 slice whole wheat bread
  1 egg white
  1 tablespoon skim milk
  1 tablespoon orange juice
  1/4 teaspoon cinnamon
  1/4 oz. chopped macadamia nuts
  1 tablespoon maple syrup
8 oz. skim milk
6 oz. hot beverage

LUNCH
Turkey sandwich:
  2 slices oatmeal bread
  2 slices turkey breast
  1 oz. provolone cheese
  1 slice tomato
  1/4 cup lettuce
1/2 cup cranberry sauce
1/2 cup vanilla pudding with diced pineapple

DINNER
Black beans and rice:
  1 cup black beans
  3/4 cup white rice
  1/2 cup chicken broth
  1/8 cup green peppers
  1/8 cup chopped onion
  1/4 teaspoon fresh garlic
  1/4 teaspoon spices
1 cup stewed tomatoes with okra and corn
Sauteed bananas:
  1/2 cup sliced bananas
  1/2 oz. sliced pecans
  1 tablespoon honey
  1 tablespoon lemon juice
  1 teaspoon cinnamon

Semi-Vegetarian Day 5

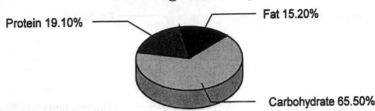

Protein 19.10% — Fat 15.20%

Carbohydrate 65.50%

BREAKFAST
1 cup sliced orange
Egg white omelette:
    3 egg whites
    1/4 cup sliced mushrooms
    1/4 cup chopped tomato
    1 teaspoon green pepper
    1 teaspoon chopped onion
    1 oz. cheddar cheese
1 English muffin toasted
1 tablespoon jam
8 oz. pineapple juice
6 oz. hot beverage

LUNCH
Pita bread pizza:
    1 pita bread
    1/4 cup sliced mushrooms
    1/4 cup chopped broccoli
    1 tablespoon green pepper
    1 tablespoon chopped onion
    2 fresh tomato slices
    1 tablespoon tomato sauce
    1 oz. part-skim mozzarella cheese
Mixed green salad:
    1 cup romaine
    1/2 cup radiccio
    1/4 cup shredded carrots
    1 tablespoon nonfat dressing
10 seedless grapes

DINNER
3 ounces roasted turkey breast
1 cup mashed potato
1/4 cup brown gravy
1 cup steamed green beans
Spinach salad:
    1 cup spinach
    1/2 cup sliced mushrooms
    1 tablespoon nonfat dressing
1 slice pumpernickel bread
1 cup watermelon chunks

Semi-Vegetarian Day 6

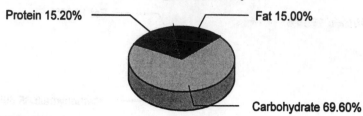

Protein 15.20%   Fat 15.00%

Carbohydrate 69.60%

BREAKFAST
1/2 cup pineapple chunks
1/2 cup orange slices
1 banana nut muffin
6 oz. lowfat strawberry yogurt
8 oz. skim milk
6 oz. hot beverage

LUNCH
Pasta salad:
    1 cup pasta
    1/4 cup pinto beans
    1/4 cup diced yellow squash
    1/8 cup chopped red and green pepper
    1 cup romaine
    1 tablespoon nonfat dressing
2 multi-grain breadsticks
3 apricot halves
1/2 oz. pistachio nuts dried and shelled

DINNER
3 ounces grilled tuna teriyaki
1 tablespoon lemon juice
1 cup oven baked potato wedges with paprika seasoning
1 cup fresh beets and beet greens steamed
1 corn muffin
1 cup sliced mango

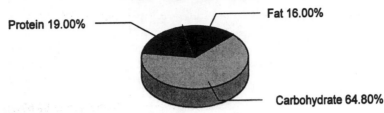

Semi-Vegetarian Day 7

Protein 19.00%

Fat 16.00%

Carbohydrate 64.80%

BREAKFAST
1/2 grapefruit
1 ounce raisin bran cereal
1/2 oz. slivered almonds
8 oz. skim milk
1 slice oatmeal bread toasted
8 oz. orange juice
6 oz. hot beverage

LUNCH
Bean burrito:
     1 flour tortilla
     1/3 cup refried beans
     1 oz. lowfat cheddar cheese
     1/2 cup lettuce
     1 tablespoon plain lowfat yogurt
     1 tablespoon salsa
Carrot sticks
1 cup fresh berries

DINNER
Shrimp fettuccini:
     2 ounces boiled shrimp
     1 cup fettuccini
     1/2 oz. grated Parmesan
     1 oz. white wine sauce
Tomato/cucumber salad:
     1/2 tomato
     6 slices cucumber
     1 tablespoon nonfat dressing
1 multi-grain roll
1 cup baked bananas with cinnamon

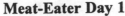

Meat-Eater Day 1

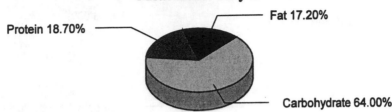

Protein 18.70%

Fat 17.20%

Carbohydrate 64.00%

BREAKFAST
1 cup blackberries
1 whole wheat English muffin toasted
1 tablespoon peanut butter
6 oz. lowfat fruit-flavored yogurt
8 oz. skim milk
6 oz. hot beverage

LUNCH
Sardine sandwich:
    2 slices of whole wheat toast
    2 ounces sardines
    1 cup lettuce
    6 slices cucumber
    1/4 cup raw onion
1 medium apple

DINNER
Arroz con pollo:
    2 ounces roasted chicken breast
    1 cup Spanish rice
    1/2 cup chicken broth
    1 tablespoon corn starch
    1/4 cup red and green pepper
    1/4 cup onion
1 corn on the cob
Mixed salad:
    1 cup romaine
    1/4 cup cauliflower florets
    2 sliced radishes
    1/2 oz. sunflower seeds dried and hulled
    1 tablespoon nonfat dressing
1 toasted tortilla
4 oz. frozen lowfat yogurt
1/2 cup strawberries

Meat-Eater Day 2

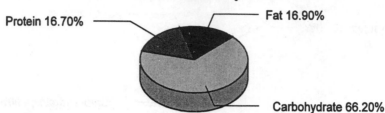

Protein 16.70% — Fat 16.90% — Carbohydrate 66.20%

BREAKFAST
1/2 cup orange slices
1 cup hot oatmeal with:
    1 tablespoon honey
    1/8 cup dried dates pitted and chopped
    1/2 oz. chopped walnuts
    1/2 green apple cored and chopped
1 slice raisin toast
8 oz. skim milk
6 oz. hot beverage

LUNCH
Roast beef sandwich:
    2 slices multi-grain bread
    2 ounces lean roast beef
    1/2 cup lettuce
    2 slices tomato
    1 slice onion
    1 teaspoon dijon mustard
Pasta salad:
    1/2 cup cooked pasta
    1/8 cup slivered mushrooms
    1 tablespoon chopped onion
    1 tablespoon nonfat ranch dressing
1/2 sliced mango and 1 sliced kiwi

DINNER
2 ounces baked flounder or sole with lemon juice
Baked potato with:
    1 tablespoon nonfat ranch dressing
    1/2 cup broccoli florets
Vegetable medley:
    1/2 yellow squash
    1/4 cup zucchini
    1/4 cup tomatoes
Endive salad:
    1 cup endive
    1/4 cup orange slices
    1 tablespoon nonfat raspberry vinaigrette
4 oz. light vanilla ice milk topped with 1/4 cup shredded coconut

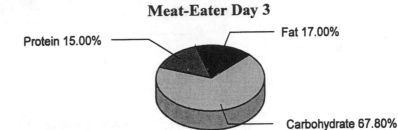

Meat-Eater Day 3

Protein 15.00%   Fat 17.00%

Carbohydrate 67.80%

BREAKFAST
1 ounce multi-bran chex cereal topped with:
    1/2 cup blueberries
    1 tablespoon brown sugar
    1 cup skim milk
1 banana nut muffin
8 oz. pineapple juice
6 oz. hot beverage

LUNCH
9.5 ounces chunky chicken vegetable soup
2 slices cracked-wheat bread
Marinated tomatoes and mushrooms:
    3/4 cup tomatoes
    1/4 cup mushrooms
    1 tablespoon nonfat vinegar dressing
1 medium-sized pear

DINNER
2.5 oz. lean flank steak marinated in Burgundy wine and grilled
1 cup homemade oven-baked potato wedges
1 cup steamed spinach
Tossed salad:
    1 cup romaine
    1/4 cup shredded carrots
    1/4 cup shredded red cabbage
    1 tablespoon nonfat vinegar dressing
1 pita bread
8 oz. sherbet (2% fat) topped with:
    1/4 cup fresh raspberries
    1/2 oz. macadamia nuts

Meat-Eater Day 4

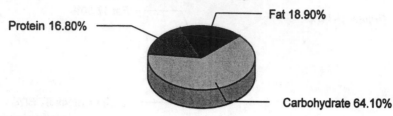

Protein 16.80%

Fat 18.90%

Carbohydrate 64.10%

BREAKFAST
1/2 cantaloupe
2 egg whites scrambled with:
    1/8 cup sliced mushrooms
    1/2 teaspoon spices
1 ounce lean ham
1 toasted pita bread
8 oz. apple juice
6 oz. hot beverage

LUNCH
4 ounces New England clam chowder
1 piece toasted pumpernickel bread
Tossed green salad:
    1 cup romaine
    1/4 cup corn
    1/4 cup broccoli florets
    1/2 oz. sunflower seeds dried and hulled
    1 tablespoon nonfat dressing
1 orange

DINNER
1 cup cooked pasta with:
    1/4 cup tomatoes
    1/4 cup eggplant
    1 oz. white wine
    1/4 cup part-skim ricotta
Vegetable medley:
    4 spears braised asparagus
    1/4 cup yellow squash
    1/8 cup red pepper
1 multi-grain dinner roll
4 oz. light vanilla ice milk with 1/4 cup sliced banana

Meat-Eater Day 5

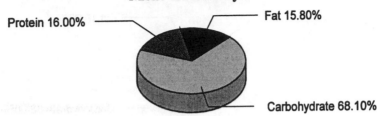

Protein 16.00%

Fat 15.80%

Carbohydrate 68.10%

BREAKFAST
1/2 grapefruit
1 toasted whole wheat raisin bagel
1/2 oz. cream cheese
8 oz. skim milk
6 oz. hot beverage

LUNCH
Grilled cheese:
    2 slices whole wheat bread
    1 oz. swiss cheese
    2 slices tomato
Apple/celery salad:
    3/4 cup sliced apple
    1/4 cup chopped celery
    1 cup lettuce
Dressing of:
    1 tablespoon lowfat yogurt
    1 tablespoon honey
    1 tablespoon lime juice
1/2 cup fruit-flavored gelatin

DINNER
Stir-fried vegetable medley with shrimp:
    2 ounces of shelled shrimp
    1/4 cup bamboo shoots
    1/4 cup snowpeas
    1/4 cup broccoli
    1/4 cup water chestnuts
1 cup steamed rice
Tossed salad:
    1 cup romaine
    1/4 cup artichoke hearts
    1 tablespoon nonfat dressing
1 cup fresh apricots with:
    1/2 oz. pecan halves
    1/4 teaspoon ginger

Meat-Eater Day 6

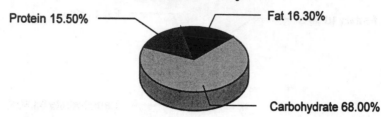

Protein 15.50% —

Fat 16.30%

Carbohydrate 68.00%

BREAKFAST
1 cup fresh raspberries
1 cup cream of wheat with:
    1-1/2 tablespoons raisins
    1/2 oz. slivered almonds
    1/2 teaspoon cinnamon
1 bran muffin with 1 tablespoon orange marmalade
8 oz. skim milk
6 oz. hot beverage

LUNCH
Crabmeat salad:
    1/2 cup crabmeat
    4 cold asparagus spears
    1 cup lettuce
    1/2 cup spinach leaves
    1 tablespoon nonfat ranch dressing
1 slice toasted oatmeal bread
1 cup apple wedges with 1/4 oz. chopped walnuts spiced with cinnamon

DINNER
Turkey marsala:
    3 ounces sliced turkey
    1 cup cooked noodles
    1/2 cup pan gravy made with wine, flour, mushrooms, and chicken broth
1/2 cup peas with lemon juice
Tossed salad:
    1 cup romaine
    1 tablespoon sprouts
    1/4 cup shredded carrots
    1/8 cup lowfat cottage cheese
    1 tablespoon nonfat dressing
1 multi-grain dinner roll
1 cup sliced peaches

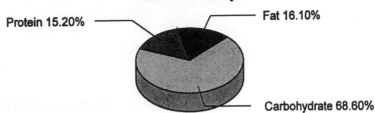

Meat-Eater Day 7

Protein 15.20%

Fat 16.10%

Carbohydrate 68.60%

BREAKFAST
2 buckwheat pancakes with:
    1 oz. lowfat yogurt
    1/2 cup sliced strawberries
    1/2 banana
8 oz. orange juice
6 oz. hot beverage

LUNCH
Broiled beef/bean burger:
    1.5 oz. lean ground beef mixed with 1 oz. pinto beans
    1 whole wheat hamburger roll
    1/4 cup bean sprouts
    2 slices tomato
    1 slice onion
    1 teaspoon dijon mustard
6 large slices cucumber
1 nectarine

DINNER
Wild rice scallop casserole:
    1 cup wild rice
    6 scallops
    1 oz. cream of mushroom soup
1/2 cup steamed green beans
Mixed salad:
    1/2 cup romaine
    1/2 cup Belgian endive
    1/2 cup tomato
    1/4 cup shredded red cabbage
    1/4 cup chopped celery
    1 tablespoon nonfat dressing
2 corn tortillas
1/2 cup vanilla pudding topped with 1-1/2 tablespoons raisins

20 Tips
for Eating Healthy
at Restaurants

- Ask that food be prepared without butter or oil.

- Use vinegar or lemon for flavoring.

- Have a plain baked potato garnished with salsa or steamed vegetables.

- Avoid creamy or oily dressings at the salad bar.

- Do not exceed 4-ounce portions of meat, chicken, or fish.

- Order lean meat braised, broiled, or grilled without fat.

- Order chicken or fish grilled, poached, or baked in wine or lemon juice.

- Ask for sauces on the side.

- Avoid foods that are fried, au gratin, or sauteed.

- Some restaurants will offer a vegetable plate or special salad even if it is not listed on the menu. Don't be afraid to ask.

- Order clear soup for an appetizer.

- Order fresh fruit or a sorbet for dessert.

- At Chinese restaurants, avoid fried rice and stir fried dishes, since they are often cooked in oil or lard.

- Avoid chowders and creamy sauces made with milk.

- Choose egg-free pasta if available.

- Order pizza without cheese, and top with vegetables and tomato sauce.

- Choose whole grain dishes, whole wheat bread, brown rice, steamed vegetables, and beans.

- Avoid movie theater popcorn that is popped in coconut oil.

- Avoid foods with cheese, avocadoes, nuts, and oils.

- Order an appetizer as your main meal. It will often be enough to satisfy.

BIBLIOGRAPHY

"The Biology and Physiology of Aging," *The Western Journal of Medicine*, December 1990.

"Can Vitamins Help?" *Consumer Reports*, January 1992.

Chopra, Deepak. *Ageless Body, Timeless Mind*, Crown Publishers, Harmony Books, 1993.

Chopra, Deepak. *Creating Health*, Houghton, Mifflin, 1991.

Chopra, Deepak. *Quantum Healing*, Bantam New Age, 1989.

"Complementary Self-Care Strategies for Healthy Aging," *Generations*, Fall 1993.

Cooper, Kenneth. *The Aerobics Way*, Bantam Books, 1977.

Douillard, John. *Body, Mind and Sport*, Harmony Books, 1994.

Eliot, Robert. *A Change of Heart: Converting Your Stresses to Strengths*, Bantam Books, 1993.

Eliot, Robert, and Dennis Breo. *Is it Worth Dying For? A Self-Assessment Program to Make Stress Work for You, Not Against You*, Bantam Books, 1989.

"Explaining Fruit Fly Longevity," *Science*, June 11, 1993.

"Good Sense, Good Health," *Sports Illustrated*, November 13, 1989.

Hewitt, James. *Teach Yourself Yoga*, NTC Publishing Group, 1993.

Hittleman, Richard. *Yoga for Health*, Ballantine Books, 1985.

"How Long Is the Human Life-Span?" *Science*, November 15, 1991.

"In Search of Methuselah: Estimating the Upper Limits to Human Longevity," *Science*, November 2, 1990.

Journal of Advancement in Medicine, Winter 1993.

Kasch, Fred W. *Adult Fitness, Principles & Practice*, Mayfield Publishers, 1968.

Kriegel, Robert, and Kriegel, Marilyn. "The C-Zone." Fawcett, 1985.

"Living Longer," *Men's Health*, Spring 1989.

Maharishi Maheesh Yogi. *Transcendental Meditation: Science of Being and Art of Living*, NAL - Dutton, 1988.

"Mighty Vitamins," *Medical World News*, January 1993.

"Mind-Survival Link Emerges From Death Data," *Science News*, November 6, 1993.

"Phenomena, Comment and Notes," *Smithsonian*, May 1990.

Portugues, Gladys, and Joyce Vedral. *Hard Bodies*, Dell Publishing, 1986.

"Protein Oxidation and Aging," *Science*, August 28, 1992.

Quillon, P., and R. M. Williams, eds. *Adjuvant Nutrition in Cancer Treatment*, Cancer Treatment Research Foundation, 1993.

Russell, Peter. *The TM Technique: An Introduction to Transcendental Meditation and the Teachings of Maharishi Maheesh Yogi*, Viking-Penguin, 1989.

Sears, Barry. "Essential Fatty Acids and Dietary Endocrinology: A Hypothesis for Cardiovascular Treatment," *The Journal of Advancement in Medicine*, Vol. 6, No. 4, Human Sciences Press Inc., 1993.

Sears, Barry. "Chapter 14: Essential Fatty Acids, Eicosanoids and Cancer," *Adjuvant Nutrition in Cancer Treatment*, edited by P. Quillon and R. M. Williams, Cancer Treatment Research Foundation, 1993.

Seyle, Hans. *Stress Without Distress*, NAL - Dutton, 1975.

Sharma, Hari. *Freedom From Disease*, Atrium Books, 1992.

"Slow Forward," *American Health: Fitness of Body and Mind*, July-August 1989.

Sprague, Ken. *The Gold's Gym Book of Weight Training*, Perigee Books, 1993.

"Survival of the Fittest," *Health*, May-June 1993.

"The Three Secrets of Shangri-La," *In Health*, July-August 1990.

"Toward a New Image of Aging," *Prevention Magazine*, June 1990.

"Unfit Survivors: Exercise as a Resource for Aging Women," *The Gerontolgist*, June 1991.

"Vitamin C Intake and Longer Life," *The Washington Post*, May 11, 1992, Sect. A, p. 2.

"The War on Aging," *Life*, October 1992.

"Why Do We Age?" *Scientific American*, December 1992.

Willix, Robert. *Keep Your Miles High and Your Calories Low*, M.M. & B. Publishing, 1990.

Willix, Robert. *Stress Management for the Business Executive* (privately published paper), 1992.

"Working Out Shapes Up to a Longer Life," *USA Today*, February 25, 1993, Sect. A, p. 2.

Zebroff, Kareen. *Back Fitness the Yoga Way*, Gordon Boules Books, 1989.

About the Author

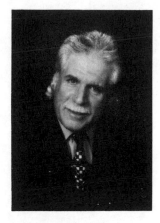

Robert D. Willix Jr. is a graduate of Boston College and the University of Missouri Medical School. He completed his internship and residency in Cardiac Surgery at the University of Michigan Medical Center.

In 1975, he founded and developed the first open heart surgery program in South Dakota. In 1981, he was recruited to direct Cardiac Rehabilitation and Human Performance for three hospitals in Fort Lauderdale, Florida. In 1987, Dr. Willix established his private medical practice, focusing on Preventive and Sports Medicine. In 1991, he became a Charter Member of the American Medical Society for Sports Medicine. He is also a Fellow of the American College of Sports Medicine.

Dr. Willix currently has his office in Boca Raton, Florida. His patients range from people with complex heart problems to those seeking counseling on nutrition and exercise. Dr. Willix recognizes the value of offering his patients alternative medicine. He is currently one of only 300 physicians in the United States trained in Ayurvedic medicine and pulse diagnosis. He actively utilizes these ancient techniques with all those patients interested in the healing power of mind-body medicine and herbs.

Dr. Willix is an avid runner and triathlete. He has completed 14 marathons and the Ironman Triathlon in Kona, Hawaii. He is the author of a national newsletter entitled "Dr. Willix's *Health & Longevity*," and editor of *Natural Health Secrets From Around the World*, a 425-page book that offers over 1,200 natural remedies for over 100 common ailments.

Postscript and Special Invitation
From Dr. Robert D. Willix, Jr. ...

Dear Reader,

Throughout this book, I have explained my seven-step program for health and longevity. I have provided you with the foundation you need to go forward and live the healthiest, happiest, longest life possible, full of energy and vitality and free from pain.

By reading this book, you have taken the first important step toward health at 100. But there is more you can do ... indeed more that you should want to do ... to add many more healthy, active years to your lifetime.

"Give Me 3 Minutes a Day,
and I Can Add Up to 10 Years to Your Life"

Do you know what I tell new patients when they come to see me?

I say, "Give me 3 minutes a day, and I can add up to 10 years to your life. Give me an average of 16 minutes a day, and I'll add as many as 15 years to your life. Give me one hour a day, and I can add 20 years or more to your life."

Obviously, these figures are based on what an average person can achieve with my program. Results may vary depending on each person's age and current state of health.

But the basic principle does not vary. This is what I help my patients to understand. And this is what I want you to understand.

You see, you can decide how healthy you will be and how long you will live. Even people who were old or in poor health have gotten well with my program.

It really is possible to feel good all the time. I mean more than just "not being sick." I mean actively feeling good. You can feel full of energy, with strong muscles, a calm stomach, bones and joints free from stiffness, fresh and glowing skin, deep, easy breathing, and, perhaps best of all, no pain.

This is important.

Freedom From Pain

How many of you suffer from chronic pain or discomfort? Headaches? Backaches? Arthritis pain? Allergies?

How many of you have come to accept the fact that you probably will spend the rest of your life suffering the pain of these ailments? How many of you have been to see physician after physician who was unable to help you? Who told you there was "nothing he could do"?

Don't believe it. And, please, whatever you do, don't resign yourself to a lifetime of pain. It doesn't have to be that way.

You really can learn how to rid your body of chronic pain. You really can take control of your own health.

My aim is to put myself out of business — by making you healthy. The happiest day of my life is when a patient doesn't need me anymore ... when he or she learns to take control of his or her own health. It's what the book you have just read is all about ... and it's what my monthly newsletter is all about as well.

The Problem With Most Doctors

I'd like to tell you a story.

In the Aug. 31 issue of the *Wall Street Journal*, there was an article that I

Over, please ...

found very telling about the medical establishment of our time.

The article dealt with 25,000 victims of a very stupid type of surgery. They all had had their jaw joints replaced with an artificial jaw that doesn't work. The manufacturer has now gone out of business and the FDA has seized all its products.

Medical experts now expect all or most of those artificial joints to break up into tiny fragments. That causes what's left of the natural jawbone to erode.

"This isn't my face," said one of the victims in the article. "I used to be real pretty."

She's now had eight operations that have left her disfigured, without jaw joints, her mouth permanently hanging open.

Alone at night, said the article, she can hardly bear the muscle spasms and the pain. "It never goes away," she said. "It's God-awful pain."

If you've never suffered from TMJ syndrome, it's hard to imagine the pain. It's as intense as a migraine headache. So it's no wonder those 25,000 people were willing to try surgery.

There's just one problem. TMJ syndrome is caused by stress. It happens to people who are so anxious, worried, and unhappy they grind their teeth in their sleep. There's nothing wrong with their jaws. There's something wrong with their lives.

The *Wall Street Journal* article said, "Compounding the surgical tragedy, new research in the Netherlands suggests that the best treatment for TMJ may be none at all, because most TMJ disorders abate in a few years."

I can do even better than that. Come to my office for an hour, and I can teach you relaxation techniques. In a couple of weeks, you can control the problem yourself. Then after you leave my office, go to a good massage therapist, and you'll be on your way to recovery.

No drugs. No surgery.

Have you ever gone to a doctor with headaches, backache, or some other problem, such as TMJ syndrome? Did he tell you about massage therapy? Or something called "biofeedback?" If not, shame on him.

Most likely, in these kinds of cases, doctors prescribe "muscle relaxants" or some other drugs. You might feel better for a few weeks, but you can't count on even that much. And for sure it won't work long term. Because, you see, you haven't addressed the real problem. You have only attempted to mask the symptoms of the problem.

Recognize the Cause

Doctors, in general, don't understand this yet. They are only now just beginning to consider the real causes of disease and to treat them, not just the symptoms.

What are the causes of disease?

Well, many of the things I've discussed already in this book. Poor nutrition. Lack of exercise. Stress and disharmony in your life. And, of course, the free radical.

I, like many other "alternative" physicians, know these things to be the true cause of every disease, ailment, pain, and discomfort you suffer. Please don't wait for mainstream physicians to catch on.

You can take advantage of this information right now ... and begin today to add decades to your life.

In my monthly newsletter, *Health & Longevity*, I explain how you can

Continued on next page ...

put the new health discoveries to work for you right now. How you can use good wholesome food ... regular nutritional supplementation ... exercise ... relaxation techniques ... and the other parts of my simple overall program to make you healthier and to help you live longer.

Medicine of the Future ... Today

If you would like to see what the medicine of the future will be like, come to my office. There's no one in the waiting room, because I don't keep people waiting. My staff and I don't wear medical "costumes," just street clothes. And I listen to people, sometimes for hours, because that's the best way to learn what makes you tick ... and to find out why maybe you're not ticking properly at the moment.

It's probably not practical for you to come to my office, however. But the next best thing is for you to subscribe to my newsletter, *Health & Longevity*. That way, I can visit you every month.

In the pages of *Health & Longevity*, you'll receive a continuous flow of the most up-to-date information about how to reverse or slow down the aging process, prevent high blood pressure, heart disease, cancer, and arthritis, raise your energy level, and improve your sex life.

You'll learn more about items I've addressed in this book: headaches, diabetes, arthritis, heart disease, allergies ....

My newsletter will also tell you, in detail, about all the other aspects of my program. In addition to supplementing your diet with antioxidants, you need also to practice healthy eating habits (I don't mean diet ... but I do guarantee you will lose weight), to get up out of your chair and move around (I don't mean exercise ... at least not in the sense you're probably thinking), and to learn to relax.

It would be too much to hit you with all of this at once. It's better to get one installment every month. (I'm a great believer in "tapering on" to a new, healthier lifestyle ... one step at a time.)

Receive 3 Bonus Reports
Just for Giving My Program a Try ...

I hope you are primed and ready to get started, If you are still a bit skeptical, I hope you'll extend me the courtesy of learning a little more about my program before making a final decision. I know it will work for you. But I want you to know it, too ... totally. And I'd like you to find out at absolutely no risk.

To help you get started, I would like to send you three bonus reports when you subscribe:

FREE BONUS #1: *The Most Important Medical Discovery of the Last 50 Years.* This report gives you the vital details of the new free radical theory of disease and aging — the most important new medical theory since Louis Pasteur's.

FREE BONUS #2: *Diet Is a Four-Letter Word.* This report links heart disease, diabetes, cancer, and other diseases to a high-fat, high-sugar, low-fiber diet. This report also reveals the "secret" to successful dieting (which is actually not to diet at all) ... and a simple, gentle way to taper on to healthy eating habits.

FREE BONUS #3: *The "I Hate to Exercise" Manual.* This special report is for people who are too busy or too tired to exercise — or just too glued to the couch to move. I propose a basic program that is incredibly

Over, please ...

simple and will take only five minutes every morning. Yet you will notice benefits within weeks!

Add it all up, and these three bonus reports give you an essential program that will gradually, easily change your life — and add to it as many as 20 years. And all three reports are yours free when you subscribe for one year to my monthly newsletter, *Health & Longevity*.

And I want you to know that you are fully protected by my no-risk guarantee. Read one, two or three issues of my newsletter. If you decide it's not for you, let me know, and I'll send you a full refund, every penny you paid — no questions asked. Even after you've received four or more issues, I'll send you a refund for all remaining issues on your subscription. In either case, the bonus reports and all issues you've received are yours to keep.

I'm not worried about sending you a refund. I'm confident that if you change just one thing about your life, you'll feel better by the third issue. I have no doubt.

You really can feel good all the time. Please, let me show you how.

Sincerely,

Robert D. Willix Jr., M.D., FASCM

P.S. There's a lot of exciting news in our editorial schedule for the coming year ...
- Prostate problems: The fate of every man over 60? I don't think so.
- The sport of the '90s. Mild weight lifting has proven benefits for people of every age up to a hundred.
- The ultimate antioxidant. A new type of treatment under study by the FDA may be a drug-free "miracle cure" for hardening of the arteries.
- Safe, herbal remedies for a whole range of problems. Migraines, smoking, PMS, cavities, pimples, high cholesterol, corns ... and much more!

In addition to special features like these, each and every issue of *Health & Longevity* carries regular departments on food supplements, exercise, diet, and ways to relax.

You receive: 3 free bonus reports ... a complete money-back guarantee ... and the change to live to be 120. I can't give you a better deal than that. I hope you'll join me and thousands of other readers.

No-Risk Introductory Subscription Offer
(For new subscribers only)

❑ **YES!** Please rush all three FREE reports and enter my one-year (12 month) introductory subscription to *Health & Longevity* for $39 (regularly $64). I understand that I may cancel anytime before the fourth issue and receive all my money back or anytime thereafter for a prorated refund on remaining issues. In either case, the reports are mine to keep.

❑ My check for $39 is enclosed. (Make checks payable to *Health & Longevity*.)
❑ Please charge my: ❑ VISA ❑ MasterCard ❑ AMEX

Card Number _____ Exp. Date _____

Name _____ Signature _____

Address _____ Daytime Phone Number _____
City, State, ZIP _____ *(For order confirmation only)*

Please return this order coupon to: *Health & Longevity*, 824 E. Baltimore St., P.O. Box 17477, Baltimore, MD 21298